S0-AGB-468

Research Strategies in Psychotherapy
by Edward S. Bordin

The Volunteer Subject
by Robert Rosenthal and Ralph L. Rosnow

Innovations in Client-Centered Therapy
by David A. Wexler and Laura North Rice

The Rorschach: A Comprehensive System, in two volumes
by John E. Exner

Theory and Practice in Behavior Therapy
by Aubrey J. Yates

Principles of Psychotherapy
by Irving B. Weiner

Psychoactive Drugs and Social Judgment. Theory and Research
edited by Kenneth Hammond and C. R. B. Joyce

Clinical Methods in Psychology
edited by Irving B. Weiner

Human Resources for Troubled Children
by Werner I. Halpern and Stanley Kissel

Hyperactivity
by Dorothea M. Ross and Sheila A. Ross

Heroin Addiction: Theory, Research, and Treatment
by Jerome J. Platt and Christina Labate

Children's Rights and the Mental Health Profession
edited by Gerald P. Koocher

The Role of the Father in Child Development
edited by Michael E. Lamb

Handbook of Behavioral Assessment
edited by Anthony R. Ciminero, Karen S. Calhoun, and Henry E. Adams

Counseling and Psychotherapy: A Behavioral Approach
by E. Lakin Phillips

Dimensions of Personality
edited by Harvey London and John E. Exner, Jr.

The Mental Health Industry: A Cultural Phenomenon
by Peter A. Magaro, Robert Gripp, David McDowell, and Ivan W. Miller III

Nonverbal Communication: The State of the Art
by Robert G. Harper, Arthur N. Wiens, and Joseph D. Matarazzo

Alcoholism and Treatment
by David J. Armor, J. Michael Polich, and Harriet B. Stambul

A Biodevelopmental Approach to Clinical Child Psychology: Cognitive Controls and Cognitive Control Theory
by Sebastiano Santostefano

Handbook of Infant Development
edited by Joy D. Osofsky

Understanding the Rape Victim: A Synthesis of Research Findings
by Sedelle Katz and Mary Ann Mazur

Childhood Pathology and Later Adjustment: The Question of Prediction
by Loretta K. Cass and Carolyn B. Thomas

Handbook of Minimal Brain Dysfunctions: A Critical View
edited by Herbert E. Rie and Ellen D. Rie

Intelligent Testing with the WISC-R
by Alan S. Kaufman

CHILDHOOD PATHOLOGY AND LATER ADJUSTMENT

CHILDHOOD PATHOLOGY AND LATER ADJUSTMENT

THE QUESTION OF PREDICTION

LORETTA K. CASS
Washington University

CAROLYN B. THOMAS
Boston College

A WILEY-INTERSCIENCE PUBLICATION

JOHN WILEY & SONS, New York • Chichester • Brisbane • Toronto

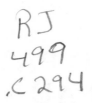
Library of Congress Cataloging in Publication Data:

Cass, Loretta K
 Childhood pathology and later adjustment.

 (Wiley series on personality processes)
 "A Wiley-Interscience publication."
 Includes bibliographical references and index.
 1. Child psychopathology—Longitudinal studies.
2. Adjustment (Psychology)—Longitudinal studies.
3. Prediction (Psychology)—Longitudinal studies.
I. Thomas, Carolyn B., 1927-   joint author II. Ti-
tle. [DNLM: 1. Affective disturbances—In infancy and
childhood—Case studies. 2. Follow-up studies.
3. Personality development—Case studies. WS350.6
C343c]

RJ499.C294   618.9′28′909   78-27230
ISBN 0-471-04553-5

To
Barbara and Judy
And Alice
With love

Series Preface

This series of books is addressed to behavioral scientists interested in the nature of human personality. Its scope should prove pertinent to personality theorists and researchers as well as to clinicians concerned with applying an understanding of personality processes to the amelioration of emotional difficulties in living. To this end, the series provides a scholarly integration of theoretical formulations, empirical data, and practical recommendations.

Six major aspects of studying and learning about human personality can be designated: personality theory, personality structure and dynamics, personality development, personality assessment, personality change, and personality adjustment. In exploring these aspects of personality, the books in the series discuss a number of distinct but related subject areas: the nature and implications of various theories of personality; personality characteristics that account for consistencies and variations in human behavior; the emergence of personality processes in children and adolescents; the use of interviewing and testing procedures to evaluate individual differences in personality; efforts to modify personality styles through psychotherapy, counseling, behavior therapy, and other methods of influence; and patterns of abnormal personality functioning that impair individual competence.

IRVING B. WEINER

Case Western Reserve University
Cleveland, Ohio

Preface

The reason for this book grew out of the achievement of an earlier long-term goal. The research project described in the center of the book was undertaken long ago to satisfy the need of two clinicians to know how the children they were seeing day in and day out in a metropolitan out-patient psychiatric clinic would turn out as they moved into adulthood. Data collection extended over two decades, and the follow-up of a sample of children seen in the early 1960s was completed in the mid-1970s. When all the data were in and analyzed, however, the results remained in the form of cold and unyielding statistics that failed to do justice to the richness of the clinical experience that went into the conceptualization of the research and the individualized, dynamic pictures of the children within their families. It seemed necessary to present the research project within the context of a theory of personality development and to evaluate the findings against the background of the authors' long clinical experience.

Working cooperatively over the last few years, we have made an effort to subject hypotheses developed over many years in clincial service to the test of research procedures and then to bring insights from our psychology and social work backgrounds to the interpretation of the findings. This combination of research effort and clinical interpretation has resulted in a book that should be useful to clinicians, researchers in personality development and psychopathology, teachers and child-care workers, and mental health program planners. The work contains a summary of personality development from a psychoanalytic viewpoint, a review of longitudinal and follow-up research, the follow-up project itself with interpretation of the results, and special sections on the history of diagnosis in children and how diagnosis and treatment relate to outcome. These latter sections are enlivened with case illustrations of troubled children whose individuality and complexity present, after all, the need for and the difficulty of this type of research. The book concludes with a discussion of the relevance of this work for mental health services to children.

LORETTA K. CASS
CAROLYN B. THOMAS

St. Louis, Missouri
Boston, Massachusetts
January 1979

Acknowledgments

The research reported as part of this book started more than twenty years ago, in 1957, when one of the authors, Loretta Cass, and a child psychiatrist, Paul Painter, were both working at the Child Guidance Clinic in the Washington University School of Medicine. They planned a follow-up of children who had been seen at the Clinic in the early 1950s, to investigate the continuity of pathology in personality development. It soon became apparent that such a study should be done prospectively, that is, by obtaining standardized and comparable data from that time on for children who would be followed later into adulthood.

Accordingly, the task of developing standard forms for data collection was undertaken. Clinic psychologists, especially Marylyn Voerg, John B. Lewis, and Loretta Cass, with their interns and with Robert Lefton as consultant, met weekly over a period of two years to devise parental forms for demographic data, developmental history, symptoms and behaviors of the child, a school report form, and a form for a record of clinical findings of each diagnostic conference.

In the ensuing years, a host of people, including parents, school teachers, professional staff, and trainees contributed time and effort to the collection of data through the use of these forms. The Clinic staff members saw to it that the data were completed on each child and his family, a tedious and time-consuming task to add to the busy clinic day.

When the follow-up itself was undertaken, some fifteen years after the beginning of standard data collection, a multiprofessional team including Doris Gilpin, Marylyn Voerg, Diane Rankin, Loretta Cass, and Janet Portell developed instruments for rating personality variables from test and interview data of childhood and adulthood.

The authors recognize and appreciate the contributions of the many who participated in the follow-up. In addition to their earlier participation in the planning and development of instruments, Marylyn Voerg, Diane Rankin, and Doris Gilpin were involved in interviewing follow-up subjects and in rating clinical data. Louetta Berger rated the children's social adjustment and assessed parental variables for the entire sample. Special appreciation is due Gail Neumann and Janet Penniman for their contribution in all phases of the follow-up. Mrs. Penniman was instrumental in locating all the subjects and enlisting their participation in the project. Mrs. Neumann interviewed, rated clinical data, and helped in its analysis. Others who did some of the interviewing were Nancy Berland, James Henning, and Arnold Mindingall. Cynthia Janes and Victor Hesselbrock, statistical consultants, participated in planning and in carrying out the analysis of the data. Credit is due the typists who are so important to the success of a research project, especially to Carol Oliver and Doris Suits.

Washington University and Boston College have been most supportive toward this research effort. Washington University, through the Chairman of the Division of Child Psychiatry, Dr. E. James Anthony, has encouraged the authors and supplied advice and space for the project. Boston College made a major contribution through granting Carolyn Thomas a sabbatical year to work on the research. Two other Boston College professors, Geraldine Conner and Alan Gordon, provided valuable consultation on data analysis and interpretation.

This project was made possible by the financial support of NIMH in Grant MH 23441 and by the generosity of the Grant Foundation which provided supplemental funds and allowed for the follow-up of subjects all across the United States.

Above all, our thanks go to the two hundred families whose willingness to provide the necessary information during the difficult days of their clinic contacts and to be interviewed later in the follow-up phase turned the hope for this research into a reality. They tolerated our inquisitiveness and gave freely to our fund of knowledge.

L. K. C.
C. B. T.

Contents

CHILDHOOD PATHOLOGY AND LATER ADJUSTMENT

CHAPTER 1

Influence of Childhood on Adult Adjustment

Every now and then, the media carry a dramatic story of crime or bizarre behavior which gains nationwide attention either because of its extreme nature or because a well-known public figure is involved as victim or perpetrator. The assassination of a president, the wholesale murder of those who are total strangers to the killer, the inappropriate sexual behavior of a public official all may set the commuter on the subway train to diagnose the behavior as "crazy" and to wonder what kind of childhood the person who would do "such a thing" must have had. Usually reporters scurry to the "crazy" person's home town to dig up his past. Sometimes these "excavations" confirm expectations of a childhood beset with problems such as dropping out of school, desertion or rejection by mother, an extremely punitive father, or abject poverty. Sometimes, however, the reporter can turn up only a childhood with nothing unusual except, perhaps, the seriousness or compliance with which the young years were lived.

The contrast in backgrounds of the participants is highlighted in those tragic events like the Mylai massacre where some servicemen went along with the order to kill and some refused and where subsequent accounts of those who participated reveal a variety of adjustment patterns in their childhoods (see, for example, Langner, 1971). Such findings cast doubt on any simplistic notion of a one-to-one relationship between a certain personality configuration and particular results in behavior.

The popular belief that it should be possible to look to childhood for the sources of adult behavior, feelings, and attitudes is not confined to extreme or dramatic incidents but is invoked rather universally to explain adult personality. Platitudes like "Giant trees from little acorns grow," "The child is father to the man" spring up in all cultures to place responsibility and even blame for adult behavior on the events of childhood. In the current debate over the use of strict discipline in rearing children, proponents of the practice claim it is a prerequisite for

1

developing "good citizens" for the future while, with equal vigor, opponents claim it has an opposite effect and propose alternative ways of promoting maturity and social responsibility.

Nor is this belief in the importance of the experiences of childhood restricted to the nonprofessional public. Personality theorists and mental health workers have assumed that most mental illnesses and behavior disorders, other than organic types, have their origins in psychological, emotional, and social maladjustment in childhood. Thus the Joint Commission on Mental Health of Children (1969, pp. 5-6) appointed by Congress to study the mental health needs of children, stated in its final report:

> We know that the basis for mental development and competence is largely established by the age of six. Yet we do not act on this knowledge. . . . This Commission proposes a shift in strategy for human development in this nation— one which will deploy our resources in the service of optimizing human development. We emphasize the critical need to concentrate our resources on the new generation and eliminate problems which later exact so high and tragic a price.

Although there is no doubt of the need to direct national attention to the mental health of children and to the prevention and treatment of childhood disorders, few researchers in this field share the confidence of the Joint Commission that we already have the necessary knowledge about the bases for "mental development and competence" from which to direct these efforts.

Two excellent reviews of follow-up studies of childhood behavior (Kohlberg et al., 1972; Robins, 1972) have appeared since the Joint Commission's work and both have raised serious questions as to the widely held belief that problems in childhood lead inevitably to problems in later life. Although there is evidence that certain disturbances such as severe antisocial childhood behavior and childhood psychosis have pathological outcomes in adulthood, research also shows that other kinds of childhood disturbances often do not persist with any regularity into adulthood.

Even within the limited context of the concern with maladjustment and/or mental illness of adults expressed by the Joint Commission, the question of the relevance of childhood to these outcomes can be posed in many different ways. Some questions have to do with the issue of continuity; for example, Do negative characteristics of childhood such as traits, symptoms, and behaviors persist into adulthood? Are the diagnosable psychiatric disorders of adulthood such as neuroses, psychoses, and character disorders preceded by like disorders in childhood? Another question has to do with prediction: What variables, of *any* kind, in childhood predict certain outcomes such as mental illness, criminal behavior, or occupational failure in adulthood?

To claim predictability, the researcher must show that children with certain symptoms, family background, life experiences, and so forth are more likely to have a particular outcome in adulthood than children *without* these particular characteristics. This question requires a more rigorous research design than that required to show continuity, one including at least the use of control groups. And even then, the question of cause and effect between childhood variables and adult outcome is left unanswered. Their relationship can be cited only in terms of statistical probability.

Most of the studies thus far have investigated one or a few kinds of childhood variables chosen from among many symptoms, behaviors, traits, family background, life events, and diagnoses. Usually those variables are chosen which can be observed and quantified.

The research reported in this book was undertaken in 1960 as a prospective study to test the assumption that maladjustment continues from childhood into adulthood but also to specify, if possible, which of the great variety of childhood variables consistently assessed and recorded at the time of clinical evaluation contribute most to this continuity or the lack of it. A group of children with an above-average incidence of maladjustment, that is, children served by a Child Guidance Clinic in a large city, were comprehensively evaluated and later followed up and their adjustment as young adults assessed. It was expected that with the wealth of information about these children and their families and the extent and quality of the diagnostic evaluations done, relationships between childhood variables and adult functioning could be spelled out. This goal was only partially realized. But the findings do, in general, lend support to other recent research, and they allow some educated guesses as to the reasons for the difficulty in showing clear relationships between childhood variables and adult outcome.

NEED FOR FOLLOW-UP RESEARCH

The urgency with which the Joint Commission on Mental Health of Children proposed a national change in strategy is understandable when one considers the statistics on the high incidence of maladjustment of various kinds in our adult population. Accurate statistics are exceedingly difficult to amass and only within the last twenty years has there been a concerted effort to do so on a nationwide basis.

In spite of the difficulties posed by poor agreement as to the definitions of various types of deviancy and limited accessibility of information, the

National Institute of Mental Health now publishes figures on those public and private inpatient and outpatient mental health facilities reporting to the Institute. These figures for 1971 (NIMH, 1973a) list about 2.5 million admissions to "organized" inpatient and outpatient services in that year and estimate that another 1 million patients were seen by private, nonreporting psychiatrists. Still uncounted, also, are patients admitted to general hospitals without separate psychiatric services. Although the NIMH "number of admissions" reflects some duplication of persons who may be readmitted within the year, the overall figure of 3.5 million is probably still quite low considering 1) the vast number of persons with mental health problems who do *not* seek services and 2) the many other services such as private psychologists, social workers, counselors, and a variety of agencies who see disturbed people.

One statistic alone is sufficient to document the seriousness of the adult mental health problem. In 1973 NIMH reported 1,718,000 "inpatient" episodes in mental health facilities in the United States, that is, residents at the beginning of that year plus the total additions during the year (NIMH, 1976). While this represented an admission rate for one year of slightly under 1% of the population at that time, the persons admitted were only a selected group of mentally ill citizens, that is, those who had come to be hospitalized. Thousands of others who needed to be hospitalized were not and millions of others had emotional and behavioral problems which resulted in conditions such as loss of or absence from employment, family conflict, alcoholism, criminal activities, and psychosomatic illnesses.

While the overall (inpatient and outpatient) number of mental health patients and facilities has increased dramatically over the last twenty years (from some 1.7 million patient-care episodes[1] in 1955 to 5.2 million episodes in 1973) this period has also witnessed a decided movement toward *outpatient* services instead of inpatient commitment (NIMH, 1976). The three-fold increase in service episodes of all kinds probably represents, at least in part, easier and earlier recognition of mental health problems and much wider acceptance of the need for help with them. Through public education, the stigma attached to mental and emotional handicaps is generally being loosened. Along with these changes has come consumer pressure for outpatient facilities where diagnostic and treatment services can intervene earlier in the course of an illness and individuals can more often remain in their homes near the facilities. Consequently, although inpatient episodes have increased from 1.2 to 1.7 million from

[1]NIMH defines "patient-care episodes" as "the number of residents in inpatient facilities at the beginning of the year (or the number of persons on the rolls of noninpatient facilities) plus the total admissions to these facilities during that year" (NIMH, 1976, p. 4).

1955 to 1973, reflecting more widespread use of mental health services in general, they now represent only 32% of the total episodes compared to 77% of the total in 1955.

RISE OF CLINICAL SERVICES FOR CHILDREN

The assumption that maladjustment continues from childhood into adulthood was at least partially responsible for the Child Guidance movement in the first decade of this century. By 1930 there were about 500 outpatient clinics for children in the United States. Until recently, most of them operated from the theoretical viewpoint of psychoanalysis which is based on a developmental approach to personality which holds that much of the adult personality is laid down in early childhood and that most of it is firmly constructed by adolescence. Treatment in these Child Guidance Clinics was largely psychoanalytic psychotherapy, an individualized therapy of the child designed to assess and to alleviate the conflicts impeding growth. This therapy was usually accompanied by casework or guidance with parents. Gradually other treatment modalities have been added, such as therapy with the family as a unit and group therapy of children, of adolescents, and of adults.

By 1963, the year when Congress passed the Community Mental Health Services Act and made funds available to the states for organizing and providing comprehensive mental health services to all, there were already in existence only about a dozen comprehensive community mental health facilities. Even in these centers, which were the "pace-setters" in that they had expanded the *range* of mental health services offered to adults, there was little service for children (Glasscote et al., 1964). Moreover, in the plan which each state was required to submit for providing comprehensive mental health services, plans for children were low on the lists.

In 1968, the Joint Information Service of the American Psychiatric Association and the National Association for Mental Health (Glasscote et al., 1972) surveyed eight of the community mental health centers which had recently been federally funded and found that only two of the eight were themselves offering any service for children, even though coverage of the whole life-span was a directive of the Community Mental Health Centers Act of 1963. This situation led, in 1971, to an amendment to the federal legislation which authorized separate sums for children's services.

When all types of mental health services to children under 18 other than those by private practitioners are considered, they accounted, in 1971, for about one fifth of the total patient-care episodes of all age groups, while about 35% of the total population in the United States were below 18 years of age (NIMH, 1973b, p. 2). Most of these 770,000 patient-care episodes were in outpatient services. That the need of services for children has only recently attracted public attention is not surprising since personality disturbance takes some time to develop in the life history of the individual and since problems in children are not likely to seem as "serious" or "dangerous" as those in adults.

When help *is* sought for children, outpatient services are clearly favored. Four fifths of the 770,000 patient-care episodes reported by NIMH for those under 18 were outpatient as compared to half and half out- and inpatient services for all age groups. There is, nevertheless, a paucity even of outpatient services for those children who need them and who might profit from minimal intervention or prevention measures applied early in the development of problems. The few surveys of serious emotional and behavior disorders in children which have been conducted put their incidence at 7 to 12% of the grade school and junior high population, depending on the definition of deviance and who assesses it (Glidewell et al., 1957; Ullman, 1952; Wickman, 1928). Although early studies such as that of Wickman in 1928 found wide discrepancy between teachers and clinicians in what they called serious problems, there has been, more recently, much greater congruence between these two groups (Bower, 1960; Glidewell et al., 1957; Mitchell, 1949). The National Institute of Mental Health estimated, using the most conservative figures from various school surveys, that 1,400,000 children under age 18 needed psychiatric care in 1966, with only about one-third this number receiving some type of help (Joint Commission, 1969, p. 4).

As the Community Mental Health Centers, numbering 206 by 1970 and 400 by 1974, have initiated and gradually increased their services to children, more emphasis has been placed on interventions other than therapy and casework, such as education of parents and teachers and consultation to various child-care agencies. The emphasis on *prevention* is even more prominent now, moreover, than in the first decade of the twentieth century. Factors other than early familial experiences have been added to the list that may contribute to emotional and behavior disorders; for example, poor physical care, inadequate nutrition, unhealthy environments, subpar schools, and lack of vocational training. The report of the Joint Commission calls attention to the need for a many faceted approach to children's problems. Child Guidance and other "freestanding" outpatient clinics still constitute over half the clinical services to children (NIMH, 1973b, p. 4) but their problems are now addressed also by other clinical facilities such as community mental health centers, residential treatment centers, school and vocational counselors, welfare and daycare workers, and many other agencies.

Psychotherapy and other forms of treatment with children are based on the hope that current suffering for the child can be alleviated and, more importantly, that more serious problems in later childhood and adulthood can be prevented. If it is possible, through follow-up research, to identify those symptoms, behaviors, and pathology that persist into adulthood and to determine what developmental, family background, and stress variables are predictive of adult maladjustment, then intervention and treatment resources can be focused on vulnerable children and on the particular conditions that render them vulnerable. As it is now, clinical services, limited as they are, go unselectively to children, many of whom would "outgrow" their difficulties without services.

CHAPTER 2

Review of Theory Relevant to the Follow-Up Study

Only in the last thirty years has there been a decided step up in research to test the assumption that emotional and behavior disorders in childhood lead to adult maladjustment. Before the 1940s, clinicians based their services to children on theories of personality development and especially those theories which subscribe to the cumulative effects of experience. The research to be reported here was based on such theory, mainly the psychoanalytic one. It was not possible, of course, to test the numerous specific hypotheses the theory generates; the study was limited to an assessment of the relationship between childhood variables of many kinds and measures of social and personal adjustment in adulthood. Nonetheless, a fairly comprehensive outline of this theory is presented in order to clarify the context in which the project to be reported here was formulated. It is followed by a review of follow-up, longitudinal, and treatment outcome research relevant to the project.

In one sense, nearly all theories of personality subscribe to the importance of childhood experience as a factor in individual personality development. These would include the learning theories, which hold that repetition and/or reinforcement of response produces persisting changes in response tendencies, as well as phenomenological and cognitive theories, which describe the gradual changes, through experience, in the way situations are perceived and conceptualized. Only a few theories, such as those of Skinner and Lewin (Sahakian, 1965), minimize the permanence of the effects of previous experience and see behavior as being situationally determined, so that how one acts in adulthood is likely to be determined more by the circumstances at that time than by any antecedents of childhood. Kurt Lewin, for example, insisted that " . . . only the present situation can influence present events" (Sahakian, p. 274). But in his formulation that behavior is a function of the person and his present environment, Lewin describes the functioning of a person influenced by previous experiences in other situations.

9

PSYCHOANALYTIC THEORY OF PERSONALITY DEVELOPMENT

Retrospective versus Prospective Orientation

The theory most identified with the premise that personality is laid down early in childhood is psychoanalysis. Since this was the Clinic's theoretical orientation in diagnosis and therapy at the time this research was begun, and since the rating scales for personality evaluation were based on analytic theory, an account of the ways in which this theory relates childhood variables to adult personality is presented here.

The history of the beginnings and the progress of psychoanalytic theory is a history of the effort to reconstruct from patients' memories, real or imagined, their early experiences and, more recently, to check the insights gained from this clinical material against actual observations and analyses of individual children over long periods of time. These two procedures embody, in essence, the retrospective and follow-up or longitudinal methods of modern day research.

From Freud's experience with analysis of adults, he formulated a theory of the development of personality which, briefly stated, is that personality is laid down early in childhood when experiences of all kinds—biological, psychological, and social—interact with a child of particular inherent capacities and weaknesses to result in an individualized personality structure more or less integrated and mature and with a set of defenses rather consistent in kind and efficiency. It is this individualized foundation in childhood which, according to Freud, accounts for differential reaction to conflict and stress in adulthood.

Several authors, including Garmezy (1971) and Kohlberg et al. (1972) point out, however, that Freud never claimed that he could *predict* from childhood to adulthood, and cite Freud's contrary belief, that is, "the chain of causation can always be recognized with certainty if we follow the line of analysis" (i.e., reconstruction), "whereas to predict it . . . is impossible" (S. Freud, 1955b, p. 168). Thus, he doubted that it would ever be possible to predict pathology even though he continued, as many clinicians still do, to have great faith in the hypotheses about patients' childhood experiences which he reconstructed (retrospectively) from his work with adults.

Freud's clinical work with *children* had been limited, of course, to his long-distance analysis of "Little Hans" through correspondence with the boy's father (S. Freud, 1955a). Freud talked to Little Hans only once. In this analysis, Freud instructed Hans' father to do the therapy with his son. Freud's interests were, as Anna Freud later pointed out, confined mainly to "the neuroses of *adult* life, their genesis, their dynamics, their relationship to normal character formation, their difference from the psychoses, etc." (A. Freud, 1972, p. 80). What he communicated to Little Hans' father as to the meaning of the boy's behavior during Hans' "infantile neurosis" was in terms of the meaning that had been gained in treating *adult* neuroses of the same general kind (e.g., phobic, hysteric).

Freud himself referred to this process as "uncovering the psychical formations, layer by layer," which then enables him "to frame certain hypotheses as to the patient's infantile sexuality; and it is in the components of the latter that he believes he has discovered the motive forces of all the neurotic symptoms of later life" (S. Freud, 1955a, p. 6). Freud was not wholly satisfied with his method. He said, almost plaintively, "Surely there must be a possibility of observing in children at first hand and in all the freshness of life the sexual impulses and wishes which we dig out so laboriously in adults from among their own debris" (p.6).

It was left to his followers, and especially to his daughter Anna and her colleagues at the Hampstead Clinic, to attempt to describe the development of personality from first-hand and *prospective* points of view and to extend the scope of theory to normal development and to pathology other than neuroses. This group drew heavily on Freud's huge store of hypotheses about personality structures, psychosexual stages, conflicts, and regression. They drew also on a growing literature in "ego psychology" from analytic theoreticians such as Hartmann, Kris, and Lowenstein, as well as psychologists such as Binet, Terman, Piaget, and Wechsler, who were interested in observing and measuring cognitive functioning as it progresses in childhood. The analytic theoreticians acknowledged the tremendous importance of Freud's reconstruction hypotheses and then set to work to study the two structures of personality he had spent less time on, the ego and superego.

Other writers, such as Klein (1939), Kanner (1943), Mahler (1963), Bowlby (1960), Fraiberg (1969), and Jacobson (1954) concentrated on the changing nature of object relationships and their relationship to ego development and to psychosexual stages. Anna Freud contributed, in addition to her leadership in the drive toward operational definition of concepts and an integration of theory in child development, a clear presentation of the mechanisms of defense in the reduction of anxiety (1942) and constructed, thereby, a bridge between the new emphasis on ego functions and her father's predilection for psychosexual stages.

Out of the prolific contributions of these and many other writers and from diagnostic and therapeutic case material of the Hampstead Clinic, a

Diagnostic Profile of child development was constructed and was published in 1962 (A. Freud, 1962). This profile brings together, in outline form, those variables on childhood which seemed to the Hampstead group to be relevant to the development of personality as a whole. It assesses "structural, dynamic, economic, genetic and adaptive data" and the interplay between these developmental lines. The profile provides operational guidelines for assessing each aspect of childhood, internal and environmental, and in so doing, represents the most nearly complete collection available of analytic hypotheses about development.

Longitudinal research at the Hampstead Clinic makes use of the diagnostic profile for repeated assessment on an individual basis supplemented, where possible, by data from the child's analysis. Because of the great investment in time and effort and the level of professional competence required in the assessment, this kind of clinical research has been limited to a few analytic groups. The insights it produces, however, may direct other researchers to the variables that are worthwhile to study. The diagnostic profile was not available at the time the study reported here was initiated (1958-1960) but the theoretical bases of the outline and its major dimensions of personality are congruent with those assessed in the research.

To review in detail the whole of child analytic theory is beyond the scope of this effort. Instead, a summary of analytic theory on child development is presented with special attention to those parts of the theory having to do with disturbances in development that may affect adult adjustment.

PERSONALITY DEVELOPMENT IN PREADOLESCENCE

Structures and Functions. Development proceeds according to changes in structure and in functions. It is a repetitive, circular process nicely described by L. K. Frank as one in which functioning changes structure and the change in structure affects subsequent functioning as the child grows toward a "steady state of maturity" (Frank, 1963, p. 31). This progression is seen, not as a consistent forward movement toward maturity, but rather as a fluctuating process described as taking two steps forward and then one step backward as trauma or conflict slows forward progress. The two "structures," ego and id, develop from an undifferentiated biological core. Each becomes known, and is, in fact, defined by its functions (Hartmann, Kris, and Lowenstein, 1946; Hartmann, 1952).

Thus the ego is said to arise and to develop through its biological (inherited) functions of adaptation and self-preservation which it carries out by perceiving, remembering, and responding. The ego develops under the influence of "environmental reality factors, i.e., as the result of 'learning'" (A. Freud, 1952, p. 46). Growth and maturity of ego functions proceed through gradual differentiation and improvement in their efficiency and through integration of separate functions with each other and into the total personality.

By contrast, the id, or sexual and aggressive drives, develops according to innate laws, and is said to be immune from environmental influences. The drives exert a powerful influence on ego functions, providing, especially in the infant, the stimulus for their activation. The hungry infant, for example, learns to search for, cry, move toward, and, finally, get the food he needs. This influence decreases gradually with the growth of ego strength and "becomes increasingly neutralized in those functions which serve exclusive reality aims, regardless of instinctual needs" (A. Freud, 1952, p. 47).

Hartmann (1950) has termed these functions "conflict-free" spheres of the ego and describes the process by which they evolve. He holds that even in their earliest forms, the ego functions, such as those of the perceptual and motor apparatus, have (primary) *autonomous* aspects, that is, they have a partly independent origin, in biological heredity, and a maturational schedule somewhat independent of that of the drives. The drives begin immediately, however, to use these ego functions as a means of securing gratification and, in the early years, the child seems to be mainly drive-propelled. Moreover, when conflict arises, such as in the intensification of aggressive drives to a degree that the ego cannot handle them, the ego functions themselves may be affected adversely so that, for example, perception is distorted by a drive such as oral-aggressiveness. The healthy ego gradually frees itself, through maturation, reality experiences (learning), and conscious effort, both from the domination of the drive as the necessary stimulus to action, that is, ego functions develop autonomy, and from the involvement in conflict, that is, they become conflict-free. (This "secondary autonomy" is discussed later in relation to the defenses.)

The ego gains in strength and gradually secures control over the drives so that they can be used in relation to the demands of reality and the welfare of the total organism, that is, in the service of the social self. This aspect of ego development is extremely important in assessing the degree of maturity at successive levels. The ego which has advanced to a position of control can, for example, withstand temporary regressions to primitive drive expression without permanent damage, and even, at times, with benefit to itself.

Development of the third structure of personality, the superego, is placed, by most analytic theorists, at the end of the oedipal period when the child identifies with the parent of the same sex and internalizes that parent's morals and values. The antecedents of this structure, however, are found in the control of the child's behavior by external (mainly parental) forces, controls which begin early in infancy. By virtue of his dependence on outside agents for the gratification of needs, the child learns, to a greater or lesser degree, to comply with parental and, later, other societal agents. He does this because he needs their support and love and fears their aggression.

Freud held that it is with the resolution of the oedipal conflict that the superego as a structure of personality emerges. When the child must give up his wishes to possess the parent of the opposite sex, because of his fear of the anger of his like-sexed parent, he does this through identifying with the latter. He takes in, that is, internalizes, the values and morals of the parent, real or idealized, and also parental aggression which is then often used against his own self when forbidden impulses again press for expression. The child now is subject to feelings of guilt when his ego acts against the superego's prohibitions. Freud knew the consequences of the acquisition of a superego: "a threatened external unhappiness—loss of love and punishment on the part of the external authority—has been exchanged for a permanent and internal unhappiness, for the tension of the sense of guilt" (S. Freud, 1961c, p. 128). Out of this acquisition of conscience comes the possibility of neurosis with its attendant suffering.

The other part of the superego, the ego ideal, is more benign in its functions. It comprises strivings toward perfection as initially copied from parents and other "heroes" and eventually internalized to be one's own ideal set of values. The self, too, becomes "idealized" for better or for worse. Maladjustment in society may result either when superego is never sufficiently developed or when the individual's ego ideals are in conflict with the values of the society in which he lives.

The development of superego depends on the concurrent development of several ego functions such as intelligence, the capacity for self-observation, judgment, and concept formation. When these functions are deficient as in severe mental retardation, superego may not develop. An overdeveloped superego, on the other hand, can have debilitating effects on ego functions which are otherwise highly developed. This is the case in some forms of obsessional neuroses.

Development as it pertains to structure consists, then, in the expression of drives according to the changing patterns of maturational stages; in the gradual control by the ego as it grows in strength through experience and as its functions become more differentiated, refined, and integrated; and, finally, in the internalization of values and morals, chiefly through identification with parents. In healthy growth, these structures develop harmoniously. An imbalance such as a too rapid progress of ego controls over id expression or the failure of ego development to keep pace with increase in drive intensity results in pathology.

Lines of Development. Part and parcel of the change toward maturity in personality structures is the accomplishment of tasks such as the child's gradual mastery of his own body, the formation of suitable object relationships, learning to deal with trauma and to cope with conflict, constructing and accepting one's own identity, and building a capacity to sublimate for inevitable frustration of drive fulfillment, a capacity which is all-important in later social adjustment.

Anna Freud (1963) discusses these "lines of development" at length and describes how ego, id, and superego functions come together as these lines cross and intertwine. An example is the interdependence of drive development and object relations. Healthy progression through psychosexual stages is dependent on the formation of object (personal) relationships appropriate to each stage of development. Thus the newborn child needs a mother to satisfy his oral needs and the feeding process provides the setting for the child's gradual awareness of a "part-object" (mother) differentiated out of an amorphous mass of his newly acquired environmental stimuli followed by a growing awareness of the mother as a whole "object" and, for better or worse, the quality of his personal relationships has been set on course. Basic trust or distrust, optimism or pessimism, and many other consequences both in internal attitudes and in capacity for relationship to others are attributed to this oral period.

Progression through the next psychosexual stage, the anal period, requires, again, interaction between the child and mother and, again, the quality of the interaction may have much to do with future personality characteristics, for example, with how willing and comfortable the child becomes in giving up or retaining what is his. At the end of this stage he should have developed his *own* control over the anal functions and taken a major stride toward his own autonomy.

Still other variables in interpersonal relationships are significant in the third, or phallic, stage of development. Having gained more and more control over his own body and the environment and having found that he can have both loving and angry feelings for the mother who is now seen as separate from self, the child is ready to form a true love relationship to another person. The first "love object" is likely to be the parent of the opposite sex, a choice which seems to arise from the arousal of sexual impulses with their biological differences as to sex. Gradually, however, the other parent, siblings, and other valued persons are included in affective relationships.

During latency, peer relationships become more available and especially desirable, partially, at least, as a way of escaping the intensity (and hopelessness) involved in the oedipal triangle of the previous stage. With a second intensification of (biological) sexual activity in adolescence, however, comes a revival of oedipal strivings. Now, however, because of actual sexual potency and the fear of incest which it engenders, the adolescent only briefly seeks after and then rejects as love object the parent of the opposite sex. The adolescent is now relatively free to transfer his affection to a peer of the opposite sex and, with the possibility of a truly reciprocal love relationship, achieves maturity in object relations.

What has just been described is only one example, and a sketchy one at that, of "normal" development in one area, object relationships. There are many other patterns of interdependence among lines of development and one criterion of healthy childhood has been the degree to which these lines progress together and harmoniously. There are wide variations, however, in individual children's conformity to this "ideal," many of which are considered to be within the limits of normalcy. Moreover, what is considered to be "normal" differs according to who is making the judgment. Some parents, for example, find highly acceptable the child who has learned strict conformity even though he is inhibited in emotional expression and in social interaction.

Conflict and Defense. As a child proceeds along these individual developmental lines and confronts all sorts of environmental forces both within and outside self, the opportunities for conflict increase. Frustrations are inevitable since needs can never be fully satisfied. Anxieties are expectable in the years when the ego is not yet strong enough, that is, has not developed its functions fully to cope with dangers, real or imagined, and when the child must still depend for survival on those toward whom, in the course of necessary frustration, he may have developed hostility.

Perhaps no aspects of childhood have received more attention for their possible impact on development than have stress and traumatic experience. Beginning with Freud's "discovery" of the occurrence of seduction in the childhood of his hysterical patients (and his later realization that the seduction was often only fantasized), psychoanalytic literature has described the effects of many stressful events such as illness and/or hospitalization of the child, separation from mother during her hospitalization, birth of siblings, moving to a new home, and so forth, and has also traced pathology to less common traumatic experiences such as the death of a parent, being sexually molested, and witnessing a tragedy such as a murder or the horrors of war. Researchers of other theoretical orientations also try to confirm the occurrence and find the adult correlates of stress and trauma in childhood in the belief that they must have pathological consequences.

Psychoanalysts have pointed out that it is exactly in an area such as this, the effects of trauma which, from the observer's viewpoint, might seem to be certain predictors of pathology, that the need for the analyst's dual approach to prediction is demonstrated, that is, observation and interpretation. Time and again the "traumatic events" reported by the child's parents or others turn out not to be traumatic at all in the child's mind or the aspect of the event that the child reacts to with fear or anxiety is not at all the one that the observer would have selected as important.

A well-known example of this discrepancy is that of children in World War II during the bombings in England. Not all children were traumatized by the air raids and those who were, often responded not to the air raids per se but to various circumstances associated with them or to the psychological meanings they held for an individual child. E. Kris (1950) and A. Freud (1958b) insist that it is only through analyzing children themselves or later when they become adults that they reveal which events were truly traumatic for them and what meanings these events held. Moreover, the significance of the event may not have been initiated at the time it occurred but may accrue from succeeding events and fantasies in the course of life. These hypotheses, if valid, may account for some findings of the lack of importance of "social history" data which are obtained second-hand and used without attention to the meaning of the events reported.

Sometimes the tasks of a new, next stage are, in themselves, more than the child can accomplish as, for example, the transition from latency into adolescence, and then he may remain fixated in his current stage. Moreover, when frustration or conflict is intense, there is often a pull to regress to an earlier, more satisfying stage, such as an earlier state or oral dependency. After such regression the child may either remain on the regressed level or, after he has gained added strength or environmental circumstances have changed, he may move on toward maturity again. When anxiety persists, he may develop symptoms such as fears, tics, or headaches and/or he may institute defenses to relieve the anxiety. A variety of defenses are available, including denial, repression, regression, reaction-formation, isolation, projection, introjection, and others and which ones the child selects and then uses repetitively are dependent on his age, the stage of his psychosexual development, his particular capacities, and the degree of reinforcement from those close to him for a particular kind of defense. For example, a bright 7-year-old may try to escape the anxiety occasioned by oedipal conflicts through intellectualization and, once having found this solution to be highly acceptable to his parents, he uses it as a regular defense without, however, actually working through the conflict.

The dynamics of initiating and maintaining defenses are of central importance to personality development since they determine individual

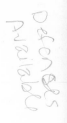

differences in response to stress once they are established. Differential diagnoses of the neuroses and, to some extent, of character disorders and psychoses, are dependent on defense manifestations (A. Freud, 1952). It is possible, also, from the nature of the defenses, to specify with some assurance at what stage of development the fixation or regression occurred that is, the more primitive the defense, such as denial, the earlier the fixation or regression. Assessment of the *efficiency* of the defenses, that is, how effectively they allay anxiety, is important to a consideration of total functioning.

Deviations from Normal Development

If adult disturbances do originate in childhood, analytic theory would trace their sources to deviations in development of structures; to impediments in forward progress through successive stages of functioning; or to regression to earlier, more primitive functioning, to imbalance among the various lines of development, or to unresolved conflicts which persist in their effects on adult adjustment. Anna Freud describes these classes of disturbances.

There are primary deficiencies of an organic nature or early deprivations which distort development and structuralization and produce retarded, defective and nontypical personalities (such as autistic children).

There are permanent regressions which, on the one hand, cause more permanent symptom formation and, on the other hand, have impoverishing effects on libido progression and crippling effects on growth. According to the location of the fixation points and the amount of ego-superego damage, the character structure or symptoms produced will be of a neurotic, psychotic or delinquent nature.

There are destructive processes at work (of organic, toxic or psychic, known or unknown origin) which have effected or are on the point of effecting, a disruption of mental growth (1962, p. 158).

Permanence vs. Impermanence of Childhood Disorders. Although she lists and discusses the many disturbances that can occur in childhood, Anna Freud cautions against the assumption that they are analogous to adult disorders of the same type and will persist over time.

Although in some cases they may be lasting, and thus the first signs of permanent pathology, in other cases they need be no more than transient appearances of stress which emerge whenever a particular phase of development makes specially high demands on a child's personality. After adaptation to that particular phase has been achieved, or when its peak has passed, these seemingly pathological appearances may disappear again without leaving much trace, or make way for others. . . . These semblances of "spontaneous cures" are the equivalent of what used to be called "outgrowing" of difficulties, a phrase which, though outmoded, is in reality still quite appropriate (1962, p. 149).

Infantile Neuroses. Anna Freud's warning is especially pertinent in regard to "infantile neurosis." Sigmund Freud had been so convinced that the origins of adult neurosis were to be found in childhood that he held that every adult neurosis is preceded by an infantile neurosis. Freud's certainty stemmed from his clinical observation that in every analysis of an adult neurosis, he had been led to the uncovering of an infantile neurosis. Moreover, Freud believed that the infantile neurosis is a *universal* stage in human development. "We know that the human child cannot successfully complete its development to the civilized stage without passing through a phase of neurosis sometimes of greater and sometimes of less distinctiveness" (S. Freud, 1961a, p. 42). However, even Freud recognized that these infantile neuroses often did not persist. ". . . Most of these infantile neuroses are overcome spontaneously in the course of growing up. . . ." (p. 43).

As Peter Blos points out, these formulations of Freud, based on retrospective data, have been challenged "by child observation, longitudinal study and child analysis, which have pointed out the diffuse and transitory nature of most infantile disturbances, as well as the fact that these are, more or less, a ubiquitous part of normal child development" (1972, p. 107). From longitudinal observation, Anna Freud supplies support for this position: ". . . there is no certainty that a particular type of infantile neurosis will prove to be the forerunner of the same type of adult neurosis. On the contrary, there is much clinical evidence which points in the opposite direction" (1965, p. 151). Several writers point to the potent effects of the maturation of the ego in latency and adolescence to alter the picture of pathology of childhood (Beres, 1971). In spite of these questions about the permanence of childhood disturbance, mental health services for children have continued to be predicated on the assumption of their permanence into adulthood.

Anna Freud (1972) has made a distinction between a true infantile neurosis (whose existence in some children she still upholds) and early "neurotic symptoms" which may or may not go on to form part of a (childhood) neurosis. In the true infantile neurosis, conflicts are between "internal" agencies, for example, instinctual wishes and superego restrictions; the danger involved is guilt, that is, the ego's fear of the superego; regression takes place from the forbidden wish to former satisfactions and the symptoms are interconnected and organized into syndromes. Obviously, superego must be present for guilt to occur and the development of true superego is usually placed at the end of the oedipal period when identification with the parent of the same sex is solidified. In transitory symptom formations, on the other hand, the conflicts may be between the wish and prohibition from the external world, the danger may be due not to guilt but to fear of the object world such as fear of punishment or loss of love; regression may not take place at all or, if it does, it may be ego-syntonic rather than conflicted and the symptoms themselves may be isolated and independent of each other.

This distinction between true infantile neurosis and isolated symptom formation is very important when one considers that diagnosis of children is often dependent on presenting symptoms with too little attention paid to whether or not they are organized into syndromes and whether or not the conflict is "internalized." Anna Freud and her group do not belittle the *importance* of childhood neurosis.

> On the one hand, we regard it as belonging to the realm of psychopathology and realize that in its excessive forms it can be severe and crippling. On the other hand, we also know that it has a regular place in the childhood of many individuals whose *future adaptation to life is successful,* and that the conflicts underlying it are normal ones (A. Freud, 1972, p. 89, emphasis added).

After all, the neuroses of childhood presuppose developmental progression through oral and anal to the phallic stage, the attainment of true object relationships and the structures for internalization of conflict, all of which are accomplishments of no small stature.

Disorders of Character Formation. Freud's intense interest in neuroses and the storehouse of theory it afforded to child analysts led them, in their early work, to concentrate on childhood neuroses and neurotic manifestations. It became apparent as they did so, however, that children displayed outcomes of stress and conflict other than neurotic anxiety, symptom formation, and/or the utilization of defense mechanisms. The conflict may be handled, instead, by the development of various kinds of personality traits and patterns of behaviors which appear to be ego-syntonic to the child and cause him little or no conscious anxiety.

"Character," in its general sense, is a universal phenomenon in man and, although it arises out of conflict, that is, out of the tension between the id and external pressures, it is not an evaluative term to be equated with pathology. The relatively permanent pattern of traits and qualities and the individualized ways of conducting oneself which are embodied in character may vary along a continuum from highly adaptive to extremely maladaptive. Pearson defines character as "reaction patterns of behavior, particularly in the sphere of morals. . . . the patterns being compromise formations [of intrapsychic conflicts]" (1949, p. 263). Fenichel agrees, defining character as "the habitual mode of bringing into harmony the tasks presented by internal demands and by the external world" (1945, p. 467).

Peter Blos (1968) reserves the term "character" for the psychic structure possible first at adolescence when ego identity is established. (A discussion of character is presented in the section on adolescence.) Before that the child develops a variety of "character traits" all designed, as defenses, to forestall anxiety even of a signal (anticipatory) kind. Instead of the development of symptoms as a consequence of anxiety, what are observable are traits that bear the hallmark of the conflict they represent, for example, oral, impulse-ridden, overly dependent or overly independent, oppositional, or overly inhibited, isolated, or sociotonic personality traits. In addition to the kinds of conflict from which they arise, the traits may represent also the type of defense the ego utilizes, for example, a "reactive character." Although character formations originate in defense against the drives, they may remain a part of the personality despite the fact that their original raison d'etre has vanished.

Character disorders, or as they should more appropriately be called, disorders of character formation in childhood, include traits that interfere with personal and social growth and/or traits that are socially unacceptable. Thus, a child with a well-established trait of compulsivity may not be able to use his creative potential for growth; the oppositional child presents a severe problem in socialization in the family and at school. Disorders of character formation are considered to be difficult to treat. Lack or paucity of anxiety is usually given as the reason and the success of therapy is said to be dependent on the induction of anxiety within the therapeutic process. In those cases where the disorder is sociotonic, for example, where delinquency is acceptable within the child's culture, treatment is doubly difficult.

Child Psychosis: Failures in Ego Development. Of all the deviations from normal development, those having to do with aberrations in structural development of the ego with resulting failures in ego functioning are the most serious in terms of overall life adjustment and in their resistance to therapeutic intervention. Anna Freud calls these "developmental failures."

Due to constitutional defects, early deprivations, lack of suitable objects, wrong environmental handling, etc., the capacity for object relatedness may remain inferior; identifications and internalizations may be weak; structuralization may be incomplete; the id-ego borders may be permeable; the ego itself may emerge from its early experience as immature, deformed, distorted, etc. (1972, p.88).

In children, these deviations are now called by many labels. At first, as was true of neurosis, a term developed for a group of adult disorders was simply applied to children presenting symptoms vaguely similar to those of the adult disorder.

This particular adult disorder, schizophrenia, is currently defined in the World Health Organization glossary as "a group of psychoses in which there is a fundamental disturbance of personality, characteristic distortion of thinking, often a sense of being controlled by alien forces, delusions which may be bizarre, disturbed perception, abnormal affect out of keeping with its real situation and autism" (Rutter, 1972, p. 320). Bleuler and Kraepelin both thought that the disease could be traced back to childhood in a small percentage of their patients. De Sanctis is given credit for recognizing childhood schizophrenia as a separate entity in 1908, an entity which he named "dementia praecocissima" and in which he included a collection of disorders such as chronic brain syndrome, mental deficiency, and schizophrenia. It was only with the study of children through actual observation and therapy that it became apparent that there are several types of ego deviations in children which differ in age of onset and in symptomatology.

From the 1940s on, one after another of these conditions has been added to the "childhood schizophrenias" and much disagreement has ensued as to the nature, etiology, and prognosis of each. Psychoanalytic theory has been applied to the several syndromes to relate each to a developmental stage from birth on, focusing mainly, but not exclusively, on the development of ego functions. The two earliest types of psychosis are related to the infant's very early need for the mother and her support during the process of ego development and differentiation. Thus, Leo Kanner in 1943 first described a syndrome which he later labeled "infantile autism." The sydrome appears in the first year of life and is characterized "by a profound withdrawal from contact with people, an obsessive desire for the preservation of sameness, a skillful and even affectionate relation to objects, the retention of an intelligent and pensive physiognomy and either mutism or the kind of language which does not seem intended to serve the purpose of interpersonal communication" (Kanner, 1952, p. 23).

Both Kanner and Eisenberg (1955) considered the child's self-isolation and his insistence on the preservation of sameness as primary to the diagnosis. Developmentally, the infant is fixated at or, less frequently, regresses to the most primitive level when he seems to make no distinction between inner and outer stimuli nor to perceive any difference between self and the inanimate environment, not even becoming aware of the mother as a representative of the outside world. Most analytic theorists no longer attribute this failure to move out of the "autistic" stage to a failure in mother-child interaction. Instead, they postulate some kind of interference, possibly of a biological, constitutional nature, in the mutual, reciprocally satisfying mother-child relationship. Goldfarb (1972) insists that this kind of defensive withdrawal behavior may be related either to organic factors or to deviant psychosocial interaction.

Mahler (1952) describes disturbances of the next developmental stage in her "symbiotic psychosis." After the (normal) autistic phase, the infant is said to become dimly aware that his needs are being satisfied from the outside world and begins, in this way, to differentiate his inner tensions (such as hunger) from this outside world. Thus begins the differentiation between ego and "other," although the mother remains, for some time, the total "outside world" with whom the infant, in his state of need, is still fused. In normal growth, as the infant of 6 to 9 months of age becomes increasingly aware of self as different from mother, he gradually disengages self from the symbiosis and achieves some sense of his own identity. When this "separation-individuation" process fails, the ego is not differentiated and a particularly severe but rare type of psychosis results wherein the child becomes panic-stricken whenever the symbiotic tie to the mother is threatened.

The analysts described still another type of childhood psychosis, more benign than autism or symbiotic psychosis and appearing later in the developmental sequence. Elisabeth Geleerd (1958) describes "borderline states" in children whose ego structures are better developed than those in autism or symbiosis but who display, nevertheless, disturbances of ego functions that must differentiate them from neurotic children. They usually use an array of neurotic-like defenses but often become extremely and diffusely anxious or completely out of control. Anna Freud and others (Rosenfeld and Sprince, 1963) trace this precarious ego functioning to a deficit in the capacity for maintaining object relationships, especially with the mother. In normal development, object (personal) relationships are formed and provide support for ego differentiation but gradually (at the end of the oedipal stage) separation from the love object occurs and allows for true individuation of self. Objects are then retained through being represented internally (introjected) and this allows for the child to function without their actual physical presence.

"Borderline" children lose the oedipal bond before it has matured. Oedipal manifestations are present in their fantasy productions but are not carried out in relationship. Having no secure internal objects on which to depend, the borderline child is often threatened, under stress, with a complete loss of identity as he regresses to primitive identification or "merging" with the object. Thus, he is said to be "on the border" between neurosis and psychosis and between mature object cathexis and primitive identification. The threat of merging leads to panic states which are one of the hallmarks of borderline children. They are beset by fears of being swallowed up or annihilated. In their theoretical formulation of this syndrome, Rosenfeld and Spince (1963) list other characteristics in terms of defects of libidinal development, impulse expression, superego, and ego functions. Reality testing is usually intact but, at times, the distinction between fantasy and reality is blurred as is, also, the distinction between self and object. The borderline child uses projection wildly and creates a world which is a frightening place in which to live.

In addition to these types of childhood psychoses, there is evidence that a few children do display, before puberty, "schizophrenia" which may be a forerunner of the adult form of the illness (see, for example, Kolvin, et al., 1971). More often, however, it occurs first at adolescence.

Increasing evidence for the multiplicity of disorders associated with failure in ego development and continuing disagreement as to their differentiation, etiology, and prognosis has led Michael Rutter (1972) to suggest that the term "childhood schizophrenia" should be discarded altogether on the basis that it is inaccurate and has outlived its usefulness. He would substitute, instead, a multiaxial approach to childhood psychosis, taking into account, in each diagnostic assessment 1) the clinical psychiatric syndrome, 2) the intellectual level, 3) any associated or etiological biological factors, and 4) any associated or etiological psychosocial factors. Separate assessment of each of these variables would do away with the confusion which now exists when children are forced into one or another label according to which of the variables a particular diagnostician chooses to emphasize.

E. James Anthony (1958) also presents a concise schema for diagnosis on the basis of several different variables. He describes three main types of childhood psychosis according to time of onset—the autism of earliest infancy, psychosis at age 3 to 5 with possible regression to autism, and psychosis appearing in middle and late childhood—and then shows how the varied opinions as to the nature and etiology of each type may be assembled on one or more of five continua, called normalcy, deficiency, organic, neurotic, and psychopathic. Disorders like Bender's autism in which psychotic functioning is said to be due to deficiencies of cognitive functioning would be placed at one extreme of the deficiency continuum, while Ekstein's "pseudo-neurotic psychosis" is placed as an extreme disturbance which has obsessional neurosis as its less serious counterpart on a "neurotic" continuum.

The value of this conceptual framework is that the child with psychosis is brought into the general framework of child development instead of being relegated to the status of "some kind of . . . evolutionary sport requiring a new psychopathology to explain his behavior" (Anthony, 1958, p. 89). The diagnosis of psychosis is indeed serious in terms of prognostic implications and, according to Anthony, is sometimes made "with a wildness and facility that is quite alarming." He offers these guidlines for a diagnosis based on symptomatology. The malfunctioning is based on:

    a)   a psychological a-genesis leading to defects in ego functioning
    b)   an a-cathexis, leading to difficulties in inter-personal relationships and displacement of affect onto things
    c)   an a-dualism, leading to confusion of self and non-self and disturbances in the perception of self. (p. 91)

It is apparent that these are disturbances in the basic essentials for the development of an adequate ego structure and, consequently, are the most likely, of all childhood disorders, to lead to adult maladjustment. Fortunately, their incidence is rare. A survey of the general population in Middlesex, England, places the numbers of infantile autism and childhood schizophrenia combined at 4.5 per 10,000, or .04 of 1%. The proportion of psychotic children of various kinds in outpatient clinics is usually less than 15% of the children seen. Although they represent a small segment even in a high risk sample of children, they require a disproportionate share of adult mental health services.

PERSONALITY DEVELOPMENT IN ADOLESCENCE

Thus far the theoretical presentation has dealt with development before adolescence. The research to be reported was designed to avoid in so far as possible the use of adolescents in the follow-up since this developmental stage is one of such flux and turmoil even in the normal child that predictions based on evaluation during adolescence are difficult. The time of follow-up of the research subjects was planned for young adulthood when the main changes of adolescence would be completed and the more "steady state of maturity" would have arrived so that the assessment at follow-up would capture what the adult adjustment was likely to be.

This goal of avoiding adolescence was not fully realized for at least two reasons. Since it was deemed necessary to include young clinic referrals (age 4 to 6 years) in the sample in order to have as much as possible of the span of childhood represented, these young children were adolescents (17-18) at follow-up. The other difficulty lies in defining the lower age limit for adulthood at a time in our culture when the usual criteria for "becoming" adult are rapidly changing, that is, leaving home, becoming economically self-sufficient, marrying, and so forth.

Analytic theoreticians had until recently avoided adolescence in much the same way. As late as 1956, Anna Freud complained that "adolescence is a neglected period, a stepchild where analytic thinking is concerned" (1958a, p. 255). This neglect was undoubtedly due in large part to Sigmund Freud's conviction that personality was laid down mainly in childhood. This belief is clearly seen in the great importance he attached to the infantile sexual stages. As Anna Freud points out, "after the discovery of an infantile sex life, the status of adolescence was reduced to that of a period of final transformations, a transition and bridge between the diffuse infantile and the genitally centered adult sexuality" (p. 256).

Investigation of adolescence from the developmental and social points of view has increased since the 1920s, slowly at first, and now with an urgency born of social upheaval in this age group. Contributions to the theory of adolescence come from many directions. Analysts such as Peter Blos (1963, 1967, 1968), Anna Freud (1958a), Aaron Esman (1975), Daniel Offer (1969), and E. James Anthony (1969, 1970) have addressed themselves to the normal transformations and pathological manifestations of adolescence; Aichhorn (1948) and Redl and Wineman (1951) have applied psychoanalytic knowledge to an understanding of the delinquent adolescent; Erikson (1956) has contributed a clear description of the psychosocial process of the formation of "ego identity," and anthropologists such as Mead (1930) and Brody (1975) explain adolescence in the context of varied cultures.

These investigations have confirmed the earlier view of adolescence as a transitional period, a period of "restructuring" of personality and of "turmoil." These terms are used in describing normal adolescence. "Adolescence constitutes by definition an interruption of peaceful growth" (A. Freud, 1958a, p. 267). It is precisely this phenomenon, that disruption and turmoil are the normal and even essential processes of adolescence, which makes it difficult to recognize true pathology at this stage, that is, pathology that can be expected to persist and affect adult adjustment in major ways.

Intensification of Drives. Most authors agree that the "turmoil" of adolescence is brought on by maturation and intensification of sexual drives which create anxiety and upset the balance between id and ego which has been attained in latency. Specifically, libidinal cathexis for oedipal and preoedipal love objects, toned down and inhibited during latency, is now reawakened under the pressure of newly acquired genital urges. What is more frightening to the adolescent is that he is now genitally potent, thus increasing the fears of his incestuous oedipal and preoedipal desires. The ego usually summons all its defenses to ward off this danger even to the extent, in some adolescents, of developing an intense "antagonism toward the instincts which surpasses in intensity anything in the way of repression which we are accustomed to see under normal conditions or in more or less severe cases of neuroses" (A. Freud, 1942, p. 167). This condition is recognizable as adolescent asceticism. In milder instances of defensiveness, the adolescent turns away from family to persons outside or to interests on which he can displace his intense libidinal cathexis.

If, instead, his defenses fail, impulses gain the upper hand and acting out occurs, usually displaced onto persons outside the family. The relationship within the family at this time may vary from one in which the adolescent lives as a "boarder" in the home, leaves home, or stays and shows extremely ambivalent feelings toward one or both parents. He may alternately love and hate them, idealize them unrealistically, and criticize them just as unrealistically, all of which represents the ebb and flow of id and defense as the adolescent tries to work through his conflict to a new balance.

The "Second Individuation" Process. Peter Blos calls the restructuring process at adolescence "the second individuation" which he defines as "the reflection of those structural changes that accompany the emotional disengagement from internalized infantile objects" (Blos, 1967, p. 164). He likens this process to the first individuation process at about age 3 when symbiotic ties with the mother are broken and object constancy is attained, that is, the mother is perceived as a concrete object separate from self and can be carried internally (i.e., in thought) rather than having always to be physically present. Biological maturation at puberty forces individuation from these internalized infantile objects, an individuation which is possible only through ego and drive regression. Blos holds that these regressions to infancy and working through the needs and trauma of childhood are "obligatory components of normal development" (p. 172). The regressive pull toward dependency, oedipal reattachments, and hostilities, constitutes much of the turmoil of early adolescence. The ego has to adopt new defenses but also must restructure itself since it will now lose the strength afforded in latency by its parental (infantile) objects. Anna Freud points out the similarity in this loss to that observable in loss of a loved one through death or the end of an adult love affair. Actually, depression is common at this stage.

The reinvolvement of ego and superego with infantile object relations is observed in many of the characteristics of adolescent behavior. "Acting out" and experimentation of various kinds reenact danger situations of childhood; idolization of famous people, usually actors, politicians, or religious leaders replaces the idealized parent; "merging" with ideas or abstractions like "peace" or "love," with or without the help of drugs, is akin to return to an undifferentiated, selfless state. When the ego is healthy enough to retain its capacity for self-observation and reality testing, it can institute defenses and prevent further or total regression. Normally the adolescent turns from his primary love objects to a stage of increased self-love, then seeks a new "family" in his peer group, sublimates his drive into "causes," work, and play, and eventually finds his own heterosexual object.

Achievement of Ego Identity and Adult Character. Erikson (1956, 1959) describes adolescence as a "psychological moratorium" or intermediary period between childhood and adulthood during which the individual subordinates his childhood identification to a new kind of identification achieved in absorbing sociability and in competitive apprenticeship with and among agemates. Erikson stresses the role of *society* in the formation of the individual's "ego identity." He must find a place for himself in some section of society and in finding it "he gains an assured sense of inner continuity and social sameness which will bridge what he was as a child and what he is about to become and will reconcile his conception of himself and his community's recognition of him" (1959, p. 111). For Erikson, "ego identity" refers at one and the same time to a sense of individual identity, to an unconscious striving for a continuity of personal character, to an ego synthesis, and to maintenance of an inner solidarity with a *group's* ideals and identity. The formation of ego identity is, to Erikson, a formidable task and he wonders how a stage as "abnormal as adolescence can be trusted to accomplish it!" (Esman, 1975, p. 191).

For Peter Blos (1968) the tasks of the second individuation and of the formation of ego identity are both part of character formation, an integrative process which he considers to be "synonymous" with adolescence. ". . . The formation of character in adolescence is the outcome of psychic restructuring or, in other words, it is the manifest sign of a completed . . . passage through adolescence" (Blos, 1968, p. 246). He differentiates this integrated end-product from the fragmentary "character traits" of childhood described previously in this chapter. Character is the *experience* of self, an experience of a stable *inner* or internalized gestalt, an experience which supplants in reliability and sameness that which the child derives from a protective environment.

Blos discusses four preconditions to the formation of (adult) character. One is the second individuation described above, which takes the adolescent through "social way stations" of new identification, that is, with friends, "the group," and so forth, to the more permanent seeking of adult object relationships. A second precondition is the "conquest of residual trauma of childhood," that is, assimilating the inevitable residues of this trauma into egosyntonic, or at least non-anxiety-producing character traits. This process is one in which the residual trauma loses the capacity to trip off signal anxiety repetitiously. Thus a traumatic separation anxiety may be divested of its cataclysmic effects even though it may be represented in character still as an acceptable part of the self, as, for example, in a tendency to dawdle at times of departure.

A third precondition of character formation is "ego continuity" or a realization of one's *past* history to achieve a sense of wholeness, which is important to identity. Many adopted children, for instance, try frantically to find their natural parents at adolescence. Blos' fourth precondition is that of sexual identity, which includes gender identity and much more. It is manifested in the adolescent's growing capacity for seeking and finding heterosexual objects but also in the absorption into *character* of the remnants of childhood bisexual residuals, as, for example, the "tenderness" observable in mature males.

Healthy character makes for an inner constancy which frees man for the creative use of potential and allows him to cope with the environment with a sense of security.

Relationship of Adolescence to Adult Pathology. Since adolescence comes at the end of childhood but comprises a "major overhaul" of the personality functioning of childhood, it is highly important in any consideration of the continuity of pathology from childhood to adulthood. During adolescence itself, disturbances of childhood may be exacerbated in the throes of the expectable turmoil. Childhood inadequacies, especially in the quality of ego strength, which have gone undetected in the relatively protected circumstances of childhood, may, under new pressures, become highly visible in adolescence. New disorders arising from the particular demands of adolescence may appear and, certainly, old (that is, childhood) disorders may decrease or disappear in the process of adolescent restructuring and maturation. Added to the difficulties these possibilities pose for the task of prediction across the bridge of adolescence is the problem of spotting "true" (i.e., persistent) pathology in the debris of expectable adolescent turmoil.

One adolescent pattern which bodes ill for adult adjustment is the solidification of character too early in development. When, with the first pubertal anxiety, the ego resists (normal) regression with its chance for working through conflicts and erects, instead, a massive defensive structure such as obsessive-compulsiveness or strict conformity, the character loses the flexibility it will surely need in facing inevitable conflicts in the future. If these conflicts are intense enough, a pervasive breakdown in ego organization may result. This may be one explanation for those instances when a very good and conforming adolescent suddenly "goes berserk."

Other types of pathology are seen in failures in the various restructuring tasks of adolescence. For example, when the second individuation fails, the regression to infantile attachments (and hostilities) may become permanent, with a concomitant failure to move ahead into mature adulthood. Depending on such other factors as the initial strength of the ego and the social circumstances, neurotic, schizoid, or even schizophrenic disorders may result.

In other cases, failure of the individuation process may result in acting out, which is, indeed, a frequent manifestation in adolescence. Blos (1963) and others (Anthony, 1970; Jacobson, 1957) describe a process in which the "disengagement from the internalized love and hate objects is accompanied by a profound sense of loss and isolation," which is followed by a turning "to the outside world, to sensory stimulation (and gratification) and to activity" (Blos, 1963, p. 125).

Given the biological ascendency of sexual and aggressive drives normal at this stage, the acting out often is sexual or aggressive and the objects of the drives are often not even seen as whole objects but only as part-objects devoid of personal significance. This depersonalization may be at the base of adolescent crimes against total strangers. Other cases of acting out seem to be attempts to reconstitute traumatic, often dimly known, past history, such as identifying with a delinquent, long-lost parent or when rape is a displacement of hostility onto other women as revenge over early desertion by a mother.

Much of the psychoanalytic theory about adolescence has been formulated from clinical experience with disturbed adolescents. Several authors (e.g., Masterson, 1968; Offer, 1969) complain that this practice has blurred the distinction between what may be quite different patterns if "normal adolescents" in turmoil were studied separately and compared with psychiatrically ill adolescents.

PROSPECTS FOR PREDICTION AND PREVENTION OF PATHOLOGY

In a presentation in 1950 which was truly remarkable in terms of foresight, Ernest Kris posed many of the questions about prediction and its logical consequence, prevention, with which researchers are struggling today. This paper, humbly entitled, "Notes on the Development and on Some Current

Problems of Psychoanalytic Child Psychology," supported the growing trend toward direct child observation and then warned that if pathology is to be prevented, "we will not only have to learn how to observe but also how and what to predict" (Kris, 1950, p. 42).

How soon can we, from observational data, predict that pathology exists in a given child; how soon can we spot it in a child's behavior, from that of the family unit, or from the history of mother and child? Which therapeutic steps are appropriate to each age level and its disturbance, or to each typical group of disturbance? The problem of diagnosis and indication requires constant refinement; the severity of one isolated symptom does not lend itself as indication for therapy. . . . The self-healing qualities of further development are little known. How much can latency, prepuberty or adolescence do to mitigate earlier deviation or to make the predisposition to such disturbances manifest? (Kris, pp. 37-38.)

Anna Freud's (1958b) response to this paper in her memorial lecture in Kris' honor repeated his conviction that prediction rests squarely on the possibility of accurate assessment and diagnosis in childhood. Like Kris, she points up the difficulties in the task: ". . . Our diagnoses usually come too late, when the disturbance has become massive and ingrained already, and the dividing line between normality and pathology is too easy to miss" (p. 96). To these practical problems in diagnosis, she adds factors in personality development that make prediction difficult: 1) the rate of maturational progress may be uneven in different aspects of development and lead to "a variety of unexpected and unpredictable deviations" (p. 98); 2) there is, as yet, no way to assess the *quantitative* factor in drive development, a factor, nevertheless, upon which conflict solutions within the personality will be determined; 3) the unpredictability of environmental happenings; and, finally, 4) the self-healing qualities of further development (pp. 97, 98).

These analysts believed that the only hope for overcoming these tremendous obstacles to prediction were "organized, systematic, longitudinal studies of a selected number of individual children supplemented and checked at various points by analytic investigation" (A. Freud, 1958b, p. 94). This intensive approach to the problem of prediction is a rare occurrence in current research efforts of longitudinal and follow-up studies.

CHAPTER 3

Review of Outcome Research With Children

When research was first undertaken to study the relationship between child and adult disorders it was, like early psychoanalysis, purely retrospective, that is, research in which the child data are not collected in childhood but are obtained from the subject or other sources during adulthood. Where such data depend on the memory of the adult subject or his contemporaries, much inaccuracy and distortion are to be expected.

Kohlberg and associates (1972) use the term "follow-back" to specify the type of retrospective study in which adults' outcomes are related to earlier childhood traits, behaviors, and symptoms through the use of *records*, such as those of schools or clinics. These studies provide more reliable childhood data than the "memory" research but, as Kohlberg points out, they yield:

. . . reliable knowledge as to *connections* between child and adult behavior [but] ordinarily cannot provide knowledge usable for individual *predictions* of adult outcome from childhood behavior. . . . Before a characteristic may be called a predictor of a given outcome, it must be shown that children with the characteristic are significantly more likely to develop the outcome than children without it. (1972, pp. 1219-20.)

In the follow-back type of study it may be shown that persons with a certain type of outcome, for example, suicides, had a high percentage of a specific childhood experience such as loss of mother, but to be *predictive* it would be necessary to show that significantly more children who lose their mothers in childhood commit suicide as adults than do children who are comparable in other ways but who have *not* lost their mothers.

Predictive studies of outcome can be done retrospectively, that is, when the subjects are adult, if 1) the data of childhood are a matter of record and 2) records of a control, or comparison, group of peers from the subject's childhood can be obtained. This is the case in the well-done and widely quoted Robins' (1966) research which was initiated thirty years after the clinic referrals of her adult subjects but which depended on clinic and school records of Child Guidance patients and school records of a control group from the same period of time. In this design, of course, the clinic group had much more

31

data available than the control group and comparisons between groups were, therefore, limited.

The follow-up research design used in the present study overcomes many of the difficulties inherent in retrospective studies. When the plan is set up during the *childhood* of the subjects, the *same* data can be collected across all children and their families. Moreover, these data can be collected in a systematic manner which assures, insofar as possible, that the data can be quantified and subjected to statistical treatment and that the later follow-up data can be similarly handled. Collecting the data in an objective, planned form in childhood also allows for *prediction* to adulthood, either for each individual child or for a group of children sharing some common characteristics.

Few studies with a follow-up planned in the childhood of the subjects have been conducted to date. Of these, the most carefully planned and rigorously conducted follow-up studies, sometimes called "follow-through," have been the longitudinal studies of "normal" children from infancy to adulthood (Baldwin, 1960; Bayley, 1940; Jones et al., 1971; Kagan and Moss, 1962; Murphy and Moriarty, 1976; Thomas et al., 1968). These studies which seek to chart normative data in various areas of development, individual differences, and factors influencing individual and group changes usually report among their findings those deviances that are "clinical" in degree. Some of the studies then look further into such deviant groups, relate childhood variables to adult outcomes, and compare these groups with their normative childhood and adult data (Livson and Peskin, 1967; Peskin, 1972; Thomas and Chess, 1976).

In addition to the time element in the designs, outcome research varies also according to the use of control groups. Most of the studies of the 1940s and 1950s had no control groups whatsoever (Bronner, 1944; Frazee, 1953; Witmer and Keller, 1942). More recently, two commonly used designs include a control measure. The first compares a deviant group, either in childhood or adult outcome, with a "normal group" which is like the deviant group in one or more important variables but not in the variable of the deviance. The second is a "high risk" design in which the whole group of subjects is considered to have a greater-than-chance likelihood of showing deviance later in life. Data are collected on all the subjects and the "control" group becomes those subjects who do *not* develop (or continue to have) the deviance in question (Mednick and McNeil, 1968).

In the study reported here the "high risk" subjects are those referred to the Washington University Child Guidance Clinic as children in 1961-1965 for a wide variety of problems. Those who were found, in 1974-1976, to have developed (or retained) various kinds of disturbance in adulthood are the experimental group, and the control group are those of the clinic patients who did not retain their disorders or develop adult disorders. Since all subjects in these two groups were administered the same forms and diagnostic procedures at the clinic, they can be compared in detail to specify differences between them in childhood data. The variable of therapeutic intervention is also taken into account.

Summary of Relevant Studies. The Kohlberg, LaCrosse, and Ricks (1972) review of the literature in this field to 1971 is excellent and comprehensive and is not repeated here. Rather, those studies are reviewed which are relevant to the particular kinds of deviance represented in our sample and those which allow for a comparison in variables, methodology, and results. The review includes both high risk and traditional control group research and proceeds from studies similar to our own in including a wide variety of childhood problems to those that are limited to one or to a few kinds of childhood disorders. The review includes, next, reports from longitudinal normative studies where deviant groups have been identified and followed. Finally, research designed to study the outcome of therapy is reviewed.

RESEARCH ON HIGH RISK CHILDREN

Studies of Multi-Diagnostic Childhood Referrals

Perhaps the study most comparable to our own in terms of subjects is that of the child guidance clinics of the Jewish Board of Guardians (Lehrman et al., 1949). Like our sample, the children were referred for a variety of behaviors and symptoms and the psychiatric diagnoses were mainly character disorders and neuroses with a few severe disorders (6% psychopathic and 7% psychotic and prepsychotic children). Since this was a short-term (one year) follow-up with its main purpose the assessment of success or failure of treatment, it is reviewed in relation to the therapy outcome research. Although all the children were at "high risk," that is, had been referred to child guidance for various problems, the "control group" as defined by these researchers was the nontreated children whose outcome was compared to the experimental or treated group.

A second study using child guidance data is that of Merrill Roff (1974). This is essentially a "follow-back" study since subjects were chosen *as adults* and included fifty each, "neurotic," "bad conduct," and "adequately adjusted" young men, so diagnosed from their military service records. This study fits the "high risk" design since only those adults were included who had been to child guidance clinics at age 12 or younger. Moreover, when the authors refer to their "control" group, they mean those men who turned out to be well-adjusted even though they, too, had been in the high risk status of child guidance referrals as children.

A rigorous system of defining parent, child, and parent-child variables was developed and the old child guidance case records were read to make judgments on lists of these items. In addition, the workers made a "global" prediction for each case record as to which of the three groups the child would be in as an adult. Prediction was quite accurate for the "bad conduct" (outcome) cases, while the "neurotic" cases and the controls were confused with one another in prediction and the neurotics, in particular, were spread over all three possible outcome predictions.

These findings were essentially in agreement with other parts of the study which found that there is a set of symptoms, behaviors, and family characteristics in the child guidance record significantly associated with the "bad conduct" outcome of adulthood. Among these are disobedience, defiance of authority, running away, and a variety of parental characteristics such as neglect, negative evaluation of the child, and inadequate parental control.

Those who turned out to be neurotic as adults were differentiated in their symptomatology and parent characteristics from these "bad-conduct" cases but were found to be quite similar to the child guidance referrals who turned out to be socially adjusted. The few childhood differences that did appear between the neurotic and adequately adjusted groups were such variables as father's nervousness, happiness in the marriage (but not broken marriages), and parental disagreement about discipline. In all, few childhood items were found to differentiate these two groups in adulthood but both were differentiated on several childhood items from the "bad-conduct" adults.

This study had the advantage of military records to assess adult adjustment but it depended on a wide variety of records from many child guidance clinics and appraisal of them years later rather than on planned and standard data collection in childhood. The records were not at all consistent as to the information they contained so that the absence of a particular item, for example, a symptom or a type of interaction between parent and child, may mean only that the worker had not covered that area in the clinic interviews rather than that this behavior had not occurred. Roff and Golden provide a scale, the CAP (Child and Parent), for rating child, parent, parent-child, and family items from case records (in Roff, 1974, pp. 143-149).

A recent study by Mellsop (1972), in Melbourne, Australia, traced individuals who had been referred in childhood to the Department of Psychiatry of the Royal Children's Hospital and who became adult patients at the Victorian Mental Health Department. Twelve percent (406) of the children referred to Royal Children's Hospital from 1945 to 1954 had already been adult patients by early 1969 (ages 25 to 40). This figure is four times the proportion (3%) of the general population admitted to the Department of Mental Health. When "subnormals" (mental retardates) were excluded, the number was still three and a third times as great as admissions from the general population. As Mellsop points out, these figures *underestimate* the incidence of morbidity in the former Children's Hospital caseload since others who have gone to private practitioners or general hospitals as adults were not counted. These figures agree with many other studies in confirming the overall "high risk" nature of children referred for psychiatric service in childhood.

The preponderance of males over females in their childhood group also agrees with most other studies; in their sample, males outnumbered females two to one both in childhood and adulthood. A control group of 332 Children's Hospital psychiatric referrals from the same period was selected and matched for age and sex with 284 of the experimental (called "cohort") group. The control group had not become patients at the Victorian Mental Health Department facilities. These two groups, cohort and controls, were compared on many childhood variables, including reason for referral, symptoms and age of onset, intellectual status, diagnosis, social class, and other family variables. The author concluded that "little of predictive value emerged" (Mellsop, 1972, p. 100).

A few comparisons did show differences in childhood characteristics of the two groups. Children diagnosed as intellectually subnormal were significantly overrepresented in the cohort group, as were *males* with personality and conduct disorders. *Females* diagnosed personality and conduct disorders were underrepresented in the unfavorable outcome group. Mellsop suggests that this latter finding may be due to the young age of the females at childhood referral (7.7 years) as compared to delinquent girls of other studies such as the Robins (1966) study where they were young adolescents. In Robins' follow-up, females referred for behavior problems and delinquency had increased incidence of psychiatric illness as adults.

In the Mellsop research, neurotic and developmental disorders in childhood did not distinguish the cohort and control groups in adulthood. The author points out that this does not mean that neurosis in childhood is *not* associated with neurosis in adulthood since this study may have missed many adult neurotics. Admission to the Mental Health Department is likely to be for more serious illnesses. The comparison of symptoms between the cohort and control groups goes along with that between diagnostic classifications. Symptoms of disturbed conduct such as aggressiveness, lying, disobedience, and cruelty were associated with a poor adult prognosis for males and relatively good prognosis for females. These findings point up the need for separate treatment of the sexes in follow-up research. If they are only considered together, the opposite effects may cancel one another.

The Mellsop study found no importance in factors like "broken home" and social class which are often assumed to be associated with poor prognosis, but their childhood sample did not include many middle and upper class children. "Attendance" (treatment) at the Children's Hospital Clinic was most frequent in the children with adaptive reactions and developmental and neurotic disorders who were also those with the best adult prognosis. The author makes no claims about the effects of therapy on outcome and in fact adds the suggestion that the children who would have the best prognosis anyway are likely to receive the most treatment.

The three studies of childhood samples which include a variety of children's disorders (that is, neurotics, personality disorders, adaptive reactions, and a variety of symptoms and behaviors) agree, in general, on the relative importance of the diagnosis of personality disorder and of antisocial behavior, especially in males, to a poor prognosis in adulthood. They point, also, to a relative paucity of other predictive childhood data.

Studies of Specific Disorders

Except for longitudinal, normative studies and a few others such as those just reviewed which include a *variety* of "high risk" childhood groups, outcome research has generally focused on one disorder or another. Researchers at the Dallas Child Guidance Clinic (D. Morris et al., 1954) have followed up "shy, withdrawn" children and a Philadelphia study (H. H. Morris et al., 1956) followed into adulthood a group who had been admitted to the Pennsylvania State Hospital for "aggressive behavior" at age 15 or younger.

The Robins study (1966) drew from a pool of referrals to a St. Louis City Child Guidance Clinic but the follow-up is weighted heavily in favor of Juvenile Court cases and other children with "antisocial behavior." Indeed, the main publication emanating from the Robins' research is subtitled, "A Sociological and Psychiatric Study of Sociopathic Personality" (Robins, 1966). Of the 524 children followed some thirty years after clinic contact, 406, or 77%, had been referred for antisocial behavior. Of all the children seen in the clinic during the six-year period from which the cases were drawn, 55 to 65% had IQs below 80 and were excluded, therefore, from the follow-up.

Coolidge et al. (1964) conducted a ten-year follow-up of 49 children referred for school phobia at age 5 to 7 years. Waldron (1976), citing the paucity of good follow-up studies of neurotic children, followed up 42 children from the Albert Einstein clinics when they were, on the average, 22 years of age.

The most frequent disorder in retrospective, follow-back, and follow-up studies is psychosis and especially schizophrenia. Probably this disorder is selected for study because it is easy to recognize and has serious effects on life functioning and researchers are eager to learn about its etiology in order to prevent it and institute early intervention.

Most early research on schizophrenia was retrospective (Edwards and Langley, 1936; Pollack et al., 1966; Schofield and Balian, 1959), but recently it has included follow-back studies (Bower, 1960; Gardner, 1967; Roff, 1976) which start with adult psychotics and then compare their childhood clinic or school records with some kind of control or other group. Still more recently, follow-up research has been undertaken, starting usually with children "at risk" for psychosis and monitoring their course to adulthood (Anthony, 1968; Mednick and Schulsinger, 1970).

The traditional child guidance case load is likely to provide only a small percentage of potential adult psychotics and some researchers have turned, instead, to sources where they may expect to find a larger proportion of at risk subjects, such as children of psychotic parents.

Outcome of Neurotic Symptomatology. In spite of Freud's emphasis on the importance of childhood neurosis, only a few studies of this type of "high risk" children are reported. One of the early studies has gained much attention because its findings do not support the popular viewpoint that shyness and withdrawal in childhood forecast serious disorders such as schizophrenia in adulthood. A group of researchers in Dallas (Michael et al., 1957) rated some 606 children referred to their child guidance clinic at 2 to 18 years of age as "internal reactors" (164), "external reactors" (268), and "mixed reactors" (174).

An early study (Morris et al., 1954) had followed a limited number (54) of the children classed as "internal reactors," that is, shy, anxious, withdrawn, and fearful children, into adulthood some 16 to 27 years later. Of the 54 subjects, 34 were interviewed at follow-up and indirect information, for example, through interviewing relatives, was obtained on 20 others. From this material both a global rating of three levels of adjustment and ratings of specific areas such as occupational adjustment, self-evaluation, and so on, were carried out. The findings were surprising in that these children had not turned out, for the most part, to be sick adults. Only two were so rated and one of these had not been hospitalized. Fifteen, or about 28%, of the total 54 had made "marginal adjustment," that is, they were getting along in vocational and social adjustment but had some problems; 37, or about 69%, were "satisfactorily adjusted" and getting along adequately or better than average.

The unexpected findings of this research stimulated the Dallas group to do a "follow-back" study from the files of Dallas and Texas state hospitals and court records to child guidance records (Michael et al., 1957). They found 10 adults who had become schizophrenic and 14 others with serious mental disorders for whom they had child guidance records. Of these adults, who averaged 35 years of age at follow-up, only one schizophrenic had been (independently) classed, from childhood records, as an "internal reactor" (introvert). Three adult schizophrenics and 8 with other mental illnesses were child "extroverts," and 6 (or 60% of the 10) schizophrenics were among the 174 (29%) child guidance cases who had been classed as "ambiverts." Another 6 childhood "ambiverts" had other serious mental illness as adults. The authors do not claim that they found all or nearly all of the clinic cases who were psychiatrically ill as adults. In fact, the number of the total child guidance sample of 606 who were located as seriously ill adults, 24 (about 4%), is low when compared to the serious adult illness found in other high risk childhood samples (at least 12%). The study's interest lies in the fact that the "introverts" of childhood were represented in the poor outcome group with a frequency much less than would be expected from their proportion in the original childhood sample.

A few researchers report the outcome of school phobia (Coolidge, 1964; Waldron, 1976; Weiss and Burke, 1970). Coolidge et al. followed 49 of these children referred at 5 to 7 years of age for clinical diagnosis. Two thirds of the children, now 12 to 22 years of age, and all but 3 of the mothers were interviewed and the adjustments of 47 are reported in three categories: 13 were progressing satisfactorily, 20 were adjusting marginally, that is, they demonstrated definite limitations in performance and life adjustment, and 14 were found to be "at a serious impasse in all areas of life" with 10 diagnosed as character disorders, 3 borderline psychotic, and 1 overtly psychotic. Almost all (47 of 49) subjects had returned to school after their clinic referral and had either graduated or were still attending high school; several were in junior college or college. Half the subjects had symptoms of various kinds including chronic apprehension about school exams, an undue number of absences with feigned illness, and overcautiousness about new situations.

Gardner (1967) traced the childhood symptomatology of adult schizophrenics and matched them with symptoms of other children also referred to the Judge Baker Clinic. She found neurotic symptoms of anxiety, phobia, obsessive traits, and hysteria were positively associated with adult schizophrenia in males but not in females. Unlike the findings in most other follow-back studies, there appeared to be no relationship between aggressive behavior in childhood and schizophrenia in adulthood.

The findings agree with those of Waldron (1976) that neurosis in childhood is followed by a significant incidence of disorders, of various *types,* in adulthood. Waldron selected 35 school phobic children from among 203 neurotic children seen at the Albert Einstein clinics in 1955-62, matched them with 35 children with other neurotic disorders as to sex, age, and age at referral, and then found 35 children, matched on these variables, who had been classmates of the clinic children. He located 91% of the 105 subjects so designated but only two thirds of them (62 in all) agreed to interviews. They averaged 22 years of age at follow-up with only three below 18 years.

Waldron found so few differences in adult ratings between the phobic subjects and those with other neuroses that he combined these two groups for comparison with the control group. According to his ratings, 75% of the former patients were *at least* mildly ill as adults as compared to only 15% of the controls; 64% of the former patients and only 15% of the control group were mildly to moderately ill, and 12% of the former patients were severely ill while none of the control group were so diagnosed. The "moderate" illnesses of adulthood included neuroses and character disorders and the serious illnesses were personality disorders and psychoses.

Waldron warns against a diagnosis based only on symptomatology. In this study, clinical evaluation agreed well with one based on symptoms for the *patient* group but there was a wide discrepancy in the control group between judgment based on symptoms (35% ill) and that based on clinical evaluation (15%, only, judged to be ill). It may be that the differences between deviant groups and "normals" are not tapped when only symptoms are used in the comparison and that this might be especially true in neuroses where less overt indices (internalized anxieties, excessive worry, etc.) are part of the (clinical) diagnosis.

Although the chief interest in the Robins study was "to describe the childhood predictors and the adult course of child guidance patients who as adults were diagnosed sociopathic personality" (Robins, 1966, p. 238), the childhood characteristics of those found to be neurotic as adults were also presented in the findings. The child guidance sample had been selected, indeed, to include enough children *without* antisocial behavior, 118 of the 524 for whom follow-up was sought, so that adult comparisons could be made between the antisocial children and those referred for other reasons. Like the antisocial children, these "other" children were not given childhood psychiatric diagnoses (labels) in the research. In adulthood, however, an attempt was made to diagnose all the follow-up subjects and it was possible to classify all but 13% of the former patients and 9% of the control group. Nineteen percent of the patient group and *25%* of the control group were judged, as adults, to be neurotic.

Robins divides these neurotics, 86 in all, into 32 with anxiety neuroses, 22 hysterics, 30 undiagnosed neurotics, and 2 depressives. She presents the findings separately for males and females since the rate of neurosis among the females was significantly higher than among males and its antecedents differed for the two sexes. Robins also singled out "hysteria" for separate treatment since it occurred *only* in female adults and its antecedents were quite different from the other neuroses. Briefly, the childhood behavior of adult hysterics resembled that of the female sociopathic personalities in many ways: incorrigible, sexual acting out, staying out late, or running away from home. The childhood antisocial behavior of the hysterics was less frequent and less serious, however, than that of those women later diagnosed as sociopathic.

Another surprising finding is that, other than for hysteria, few differences were found between the childhood histories of expatients diagnosed neurotic and those of *well* adults. "For neither the men nor the women would the childhood information available about behavior problems or family inadequacies have permitted predicting who would be neurotic and who well as adults" (p. 256). For girls, the overall level of antisocial symptoms was the same for those later diagnosed neurotic or well and no other symptoms significantly differentiated the two groups. For boys, among those later diagnosed as neurotic the only significant difference in symptoms was that they had eating problems more often than patients later found to be well. These "well" adult males had more antisocial behavior as children than the preneurotics but the difference was not significant.

Robins suggests that neurotics "display their initial symptoms after age 13 or 14, the age by which most children had been referred to the clinic . . . Apparently then, whatever brought these children to a child guidance clinic does not seem related to their adult diagnosis as neurotic" (p. 256).

Outcome of Antisocial Behavior. Evidence is accumulating as to the importance of severe antisocial acting out behavior in childhood as an antecedent to serious kinds of maladjustment in adulthood. Early studies in juvenile delinquency such as those of Healy and Bronner (1936) and the Gluecks (1940, 1959) at the Judge Baker Guidance Center in Boston point to the predictive relationship between delinquency in childhood and delinquency in adulthood. The Gluecks present the convincing figure that 80% of a group of boys who had been arrested between ages 9 to 17 for burglary, robbery, or larceny were arrested at least once during the next eight-year period (ages 17 to 25) and 34% of them had been arrested at least once a year. This figure was reduced to 60% arrested in the next six-year period (ages 23 to 31) and 19% arrested at least once a year during those ages. Bronner points to the encouraging results of treatment at Judge Baker with only about 17.5% of 650 children who had been treated there being classed as "failures" in terms of continuation of delinquency and "personality" problems five to eight years later. Nevertheless, many of those who had failed even *with* treatment were those with "severe personality problems" in childhood. Even those diagnosed as having "psychotic or prepsychotic symptoms" in childhood had much better outcomes after treatment than did those with personality disorders.

Morris, Escoll, and Wexler (1956) followed a group of children who had been admitted as inpatients to the Pennsylvania State Hospital for "aggressive behavior," that is, they presented at least four of these symptoms: repeated truancy, stealing or purposeful lying, cruelty, disobedience, marked restlessness or distractability, wanton destructiveness, and severe tantrums. Their median age during hospitalization was 10 years and all were under 15; 39 of the children had individual therapy while in the hospital. Sixty-six of the children could be found at 18 years of age and a high number, 12, had court records. Twelve were psychotic even though none had been so diagnosed as children. Of the 66, only 15 were adjusting well. Of the 39 who, while not psychotic, had never adjusted adequately, 11 had spent most of their time between discharge from the Pennsylvania State Hospital and the follow-up in other hospitals.

An unpublished study by Field (1969) confirms these findings of the importance of antisocial, acting out behavior in childhood. Field reports a high relationship between antisocial behavior in child guidance referrals and arrests and diagnosis of "character disorders" in adulthood.

The Robins study (1966) is undoubtedly the most comprehensive and intensive follow-up study of antisocial children to date. Of her total sample of 524 children selected from a much larger number referred to a city child guidance clinic between 1924 and 1929, the great majority (73%, or 406 children) were referred for antisocial behavior of various kinds and the other 118 children were referred for all other reasons, among which were learning and speech problems, insomnia, enuresis, excessive daydreaming, and nervousness. Of the referrals 45% were from Juvenile Court and over a third of the 406 children were appearing or had appeared before the court.

The Robins study is one of the few studies to employ a true control group, that is, a group of 100 children drawn from public school records of the same period in time and matched with the patient group insofar as possible on variables of race, age, sex, IQ, and socioeconomic status but without evidence of serious behavior problems in childhood. These individuals were found and interviewed some thirty years later in the same way as were the former clinic children. The follow-up interviews covered over 200 items of information included in detailed social, medical, and psychiatric histories. In addition, a vast amount of information was retrieved from records of various kinds such as hospital, court, employment, and service files.

The Robins findings are especially clear in regard to the childhood antecedents of sociopathic personality in adulthood. "Of all the children referred for antisocial behavior, 28% were later diagnosed sociopathic personality. Of those referred for other reasons, only 4% were diagnosed sociopathic personality" (p. 136).

Robins found that both the number of antisocial symptoms a child had as well as the number and seriousness of episodes of antisocial behavior reported were related to the diagnosis of sociopathy in adulthood. For example, no child without frequent and serious antisocial behavior became a sociopathic adult (p. 146) whereas 37% of those with frequent (4 or more episodes) and serious (arrestable) antisocial behavior were so diagnosed as adults. Even among those adults with disturbances *other* than sociopathic personality, schizophrenia, neurosis, alcoholism, and so on, those who had many juvenile antisocial symptoms had more *adult* antisocial symptoms than did those with little antisocial behavior in childhood. These findings led Robins to conclude that "antisocial behavior in childhood, then, not only predicts sociopathic personality, but it also predicts which schizophrenics will show antisocial behavior . . ." (p. 147).

Most of the studies on sociopathic personality and serious antisocial behavior in adulthood make a clear distinction between *serious* and *frequent* antisocial behavior and the more widespread, less serious and less frequent antisocial behaviors. Kohlberg et al. differentiate between the predictive capability of these two sets of antecedents:

> While this and other evidence is not clear-cut, they suggest a most meaningful distinction between various forms of antisocial behavior is not psychological but legal. . . . Except for pathological lying, nonlegal forms of antisocial behavior were not specifically predictive to sociopathic or criminal outcome but were also common in other forms of maladjustment. While 30 per cent of children with forms of behavior leading to arrest became adult sociopaths, only 5 per cent with other forms of antisocial behavior became sociopaths (1972, p. 1252).

It must be remembered that the Robins study included many court referrals, as did the Judge Baker studies; the Morris, Escoll, and Wexler study followed children who had been *hospitalized* for aggressive behavior. Child guidance clinics do not, as a rule, serve such large numbers of children with severe and/or "arrestable" antisocial behavior.

The relationship between severe antisocial behavior in childhood and the same syndrome in adulthood is, then, well supported by research evidence. There is also some evidence that antisocial acting out behavior in childhood was more common among adult psychotics of certain kinds than in comparison groups composed of normals and neurotics.

A study by Watt et al. (1970) points up the importance of the variable of sex in antecedents of schizophrenia. They used a follow-back design to match 30 nonmigratory adults first hospitalized for schizophrenia at ages 18 to 31 with 90 controls graduated in the same year from the same high school who were not found in the hospital records of their state up to the date of the study. The schizophrenics and controls had elementary, junior high, and high school records with much information including demographic data, yearly comments by teachers, scholastic performance, personal characteristics, attendance records, and social and vocational activities. The high school record contained, also, eight rating scales of personality traits filled in independently by teachers when each child was in the 10th and 11th grades. These rich childhood data were analyzed and coded by "blind" researchers.

Watt et al. concluded that the preschizophrenic boys "show primary evidence of unsocialized aggression and secondary evidence of internal conflict and overinhibition, with a substantial component of emotional depression" (1970, p. 655). The two factors (of six) which significantly differentiated preschizophrenic boys from their controls were disagreeableness and emotional instability. The first factor is roughly congruent to the "unsocialized aggressive" pattern described by several authors and includes, in this study, irritability, aggressiveness, negativism, and defiance of authority.

The pattern differentiating the preschizophrenic and control *girls,* however, was quite different. It corresponds, roughly, to the "overinhibited" personality pattern and included specific differentiating characteristics such as *more* academic initiative, *less* undependable, *less* nervous, more insecure, and more emotionally immature, participated less in groups, were more shy and less negativistic than the matched control girls.

Overall, 9, or 52%, of the 17 preschizophrenic boys had records of irritable, aggressive, defiant behavior while this behavior was recorded for only 16% of the matched controls. The overinhibited pattern characterized 5, or 38%, of the 13 preschizophrenic girls and only 5 of 39, or 13%, of the control girls. Overinhibition was a less powerful discriminant for girls than was the unsocialized aggression pattern for boys. The authors warn that this difference in predictability may be related to teachers' tendency to record comments more frequently on aggressive behavior, especially in boys, and to ignore or consider less seriously their shyness and withdrawal. This suggestion is in line with Wickman's early study (1928) of teachers' attitudes toward children's behavior.

A study by Bower and Shellhammer (1960), which is similar to the Watt study in that it followed young adults back from hospitalization for schizophrenia to high school and then matched them with a schoolmate control, found quite a different pattern for the preschizophrenic males in high school. They were rated from their records and from teachers' memory of them as being more *passive* toward others and toward the school environment. Sixteen of 20 items describing behavior differentiated the two groups at the .05 level of significance or better. These preschizophrenic males were characterized in high school as being more apathetic, careless, dependent, irresponsible, depressed, and submissive than their classmates.

Kohlberg et al. (1972) point to the danger in using statistics from followback studies for predictive purposes. For example, since adult psychosis is such a rare disease and acting out (and to a lesser degree, withdrawn) behavior in children is rather common, it is possible to find either of these antecedents in the records of psychotic adults without either being related *predictively* to psychosis. Only through longitudinal, *follow-up* research, according to these authors, can the question of predictability be scientifically approached.

Outcome of Childhood Psychosis and Borderline Psychosis. Although the psychoses of early childhood are so rare that they have little overall significance in the follow-up results of the usual outpatient child guidance caseload, they are reviewed here to point up the advantage of research over theorizing even in a type of disorder which is, comparatively, easy to identify and which should, on theoretical grounds, lead directly into adult disorders of comparable severity, that is, the schizophrenias. While they do, indeed, have poor outcome in adulthood, the great majority of these most serious of childhood disorders are evidently not on a continuum with the adult form of schizophrenia.

The foregoing presentation of research on the outcome of neurosis and antisocial behaviors in children includes several studies in which these symptoms and behaviors were found excessively in children who became psychotic adults. Offord and Cross (1969) present an excellent review of research up to 1969 on behavioral antecedents of adult schizophrenia. With few exceptions, this has been follow-back or retrospective research. In general, it shows that, contrary to expectations, severe withdrawal in child guidance referrals has not been a predictor of adult psychosis while schizophrenic adults did show, as children, both antisocial and sullen, passive behavior, had poor peer relations, and achieved poorly in school. These precursor variables are not *specific* to adult psychosis, however, since they have been found, also, as precursors of other adult disorders, especially sociopathy.

Offord and Cross point out, moreover, that a distinction must be made between those studies that use a "control group" of other disturbed children, such as child guidance referrals who did not become schizophrenic as adults, and the studies with a control group of "normal" children (e.g., classmates). From their review of both kinds of studies, these authors conclude that "the studies of child guidance populations deal with samples which, in general, are the more severe portion of the disturbed preschizophrenics and represent only a small segment of future hospitalized schizophrenics" (p. 276).

From the studies based on school samples, Offord and Cross present evidence that the preschizophrenic tends toward shyness and passivity "when not preselected by his attendance at a child guidance clinic." The studies also show that not more than 50% of the total population of hospitalized schizophrenics were identified as disturbed in childhood. A review such as this points out the importance of careful attention to experimental and control characteristics before generalizing from research findings.

The evidence for genetic and biological bases of adult psychosis has been somewhat more promising. In one of the rare anterospective studies carried out to date, Mednick and Schulsinger (1970) matched children "at risk" because they have a schizophrenic mother with a control group of children whose mother is not schizophrenic. "Over ten per cent of the 'high risk' group of adolescents had become psychotic by late adolescence as compared with less than one per cent of the control group" (Kohlberg, 1972, p. 1268). The latter figure is consistent with the incidence of psychosis in the general population. Moreover, 70% of those who did break down had birth injuries or other perinatal complications as compared to 15% of the "well-outcome" group, also born of schizophrenic mothers.

Mednick and Schulsinger relate these findings to other findings of differences in physiological measures, such as galvanic skin responses, which are consistent with recent biological research on adult schizophrenics relating two types of schizophrenia to two different patterns of brain damage. The Mednick and Schulsinger report presents rather convincing evidence for the genetic-biological basis of psychosis in a majority of their "breakdown" subjects.

It might be expected that when psychosis is already present in childhood it would continue into adulthood. The investigation of the outcome of a group of disorders in children, so rare and so severe that they cannot escape attention, was hampered, initially, by the belief that they must simply be early manifestations of adult schizophrenia. For many years after the adult disorder was identified, the general term "childhood schizophrenia" was applied to several deviations of ego development and early breakdown in ego functioning. This line of thinking was challenged when closer observation of such children in the psychotherapeutic situation revealed a variety of infantile and early childhood syndromes which did not conform to the syndromes of adult schizophrenias and when follow-up research, with only one major exception, showed that the majority of these "atypical" children did not, as adults, present the typical picture of adult schizophrenia.

The follow-up studies, thus far, have been concerned mainly with infantile autism, regressive (symbiotic) psychosis, and chronic brain syndrome with psychosis. Because these disorders are rare, the research projects have taken place in centers devoted to their treatment and study. Although in outpatient clinics there are more referrals of borderline psychosis than of other types of psychosis, the borderline children still represent a small proportion of the total clinic referrals and have been virtually neglected in follow-up studies.

Lauretta Bender (1969), who is identified with the viewpoint that "childhood schizophrenia" has a primary biological basis within the functioning of the central nervous system, has followed some 120 children after their diagnosis at Bellevue Hospital in New York. Her claim that true schizophrenia does occur in childhood because most of these children continued to be diagnosed schizophrenic at ages 11 to 20 has been widely challenged on the grounds that children were included in her sample who would be classified as organic and/or retarded by other diagnosticians and that the follow-up evaluations were contaminated by knowledge of the earlier diagnosis.

Several projects have focused on "infantile psychosis" as their main interest and all of them report poor outcome for this disorder which is characterized by early onset (the first thirty months of life), profound isolation, and intense need for the preservation of sameness. Kanner and Eisenberg (1955) of Johns Hopkins followed 42 autistic children at an average of eight and a half years after their original diagnosis. Of the 42 (now averaging 14 years of age), 23 had speech at follow-up and 19 did not. Only one of the 19 mute children had come out of his autistic shell enough to go to public school. All the others were in institutions or were kept at home and were completely dependent. Even the 23 speaking children had poor outcomes when compared to other disturbed children. Ten, or 43%, were found either in an institution or remaining at home although their functioning was still distinguishable from the demented level of the mute children. Most of the other 13 were attending elementary or high school and three had graduated from high school and gone on for further education. All of these adolescents and young adults were isolated, strange people whose main relationships were still to objects rather than to people and whose contact with reality was tenuous.

In a later, enlarged sample of 63 children in the Johns Hopkins project, Eisenberg (1957) found only 3 who could be classified as having a "good" outcome on a 3-point scale with 14 children classed as "fair" and 46 as "poor." Again, the ability to speak made a great difference; only *one* child of the nonspeaking group achieved even a fair adjustment while half of the 32 speaking children rate in the good and fair categories. Interesting and important to the issue of whether or not infantile psychosis is a precursor of adult schizophrenia is the finding that at follow-up, none of the children showed hallucination or paranoid ideas. Many of them were less isolated than they were in early childhood.

The importance of the speech factor is one of the considerations that has prompted Michael Rutter to suggest that "autism develops on the basis of a central disorder of cognition which involves the impairment of both the comprehension of language and deficits in the utilization of language or conceptual skills in thinking" (Rutter, 1972, p. 329). He believes that the failure to speak results from this basic impairment in language functions rather than from a lack of motivation and cites the failure of speech to develop even when autism is diminished.

Rutter et al. (1968) included autistic children as one of their groups in follow-up research at the Maudsley Hospital in London. In addition to an unusually detailed account of the characteristics at initial contact and at follow-up some 5 to 15 years later, Rutter's design includes a type of control group which allows for valuable insights into the effects of variables such as intelligence, possible organicity, and the availability of language on outcome. Rutter took 63 prepubertal children from the Maudsley records with the unequivocal diagnosis of child psychosis, schizophrenic syndrome of childhood, infantile autism, or "any synonym" of these and matched them on age, sex, and IQ with a control group who were also severely handicapped patients but who had no psychotic diagnosis of any kind. The control group included children with "probable disease of the brain" including epilepsy, and others with antisocial conduct, neuroses, hyperkinesis, and "other disorders." Most importantly, the psychotic and nonpsychotic groups were *both* of inferior intelligence; the average IQ of the psychotic group was 62.5, of the control group 60.4. Although the range of IQs included those from 91 to 120, only 6 psychotic children tested in this range. The ratio of boys and girls with psychosis was 4:1 and the onset of their illness was early, with only 3 of 63 having an onset after 3 years of age. Although the diagnosis of "psychosis" was meant to include all kinds of childhood psychoses, the actual sample included only infantile and regressive (symbiotic) psychosis.

With the variable of intelligence controlled, the psychotic and control groups shared many of the same characteristics. For example, they did not differ significantly in withdrawal, echolalia, lack of responses to painful stimuli, hyperkinesis, anxiety, aggression, and temper. There were, however, significant differences in 22 of the 34 comparison variables and these included the psychotics' poor relationship to peers, autistic isolation, lack of speech at 5 years, at some time considered to be deaf, excessive response to sound, abnormal attachment and preoccupation, resistance to change, and obsessional phenomena. The last four symptoms were found to be especially discriminatory. Important, also, to the issue of a genetic basis for childhood psychosis was the finding that none of the parents nor the siblings of the psychotic children had been diagnosed as psychotic.

The findings as to possible organicity are equally surprising. All 63 psychotic children and 61 of the controls were seen at follow-up, at an average age of 15 years 7 months and average elapsed time of 9 years 8 months. Although none of the psychotic children had shown unequivocal abnormality on the neurological examination when diagnosed on admission and only 2 had shown equivocal but satisfactory evidence of brain disorder, between admission and follow-up at least 18 children of the 63 (just over a fourth) showed evidence of brain damage. Twelve of the 18 had developed "fits," usually in early adolescence and associated with regression in speech, and an additional 6 children had EEG's suggestive of brain damage. Moreover, 29 of the 32 children who had no speech at 5 years of age were still without useful speech at follow-up and another 24 had a "mechanical" tone.

In both the psychotic and control groups, one-third were in long-stay hospitals at follow-up. Thirty percent of the control group and only 14% of the psychotic children had made a "normal" or "good" social adjustment while 61% of the psychotic and only 36% of the controls were rated "poor" or "very poor" at follow-up.

It is evident from these findings that *both* groups were disturbed initially and at follow-up compared to the general population. The main differences between the two groups were in employment ratios and in social relationships. Only 2 of the 38 psychotic children who were over age 16 at follow-up had paying jobs while 12 of the 36 controls over 16 were employed. All the psychotic children had marked difficulty in relationships with other people and in a fourth to a third this difficulty had remained at about the same level as it was in early childhood. The abnormality had become less autistic in over half the psychotic children at follow-up. Most (all but 5) children had ceased their physical withdrawal from people but still had few friends. They lacked empathy, related on a shallow level and used poor judgment in what they said. Their ritualistic behavior often remained but in a more complex form while other abnormalities such as morbid attachments, collecting unusual items, and resistance to change had decreased. Even the 9 children rated in the "good" adjustment category showed "some oddities." *No* psychotic child had, at follow-up, shown mature sex interests and only a few showed *any* interest in the opposite sex. As was true of the Eisenberg children, no child, on follow-up, had delusions or hallucinations.

Rutter lists four variables as important to outcome in this psychotic group of children: IQ, speech, severity of the disorder, and amount of schooling. Of these, IQ was the best indicator of all. The "very poor" outcome group had a mean IQ of 45 on initial testing (of those testable) compared to an IQ of 83 for the "good adjustment" group. The untestable child had an especially poor prognosis.

Rutter concludes from this research that the psychotic child's speech and intellectual difficulties cannot be said to be secondary to autistic withdrawal. Even when the children ceased to be autistic, they did not show improvement in intellectual function and speech. He does not, however, subscribe to the theory that early childhood psychosis is merely a manifestation of organic brain disease or damage. Although he saw evidence for organicity in those children who developed epileptic fits in adolescence or showed other identifiable biological conditions, he concludes that "what is likely, however, in view of the very variable outcome and the very variable neurological findings, is that biologically speaking the underlying pathology will prove to be quite heterogeneous" (Rutter, 1972, p. 331). Moreover, while he holds that psychogenic factors play no *essential* role in the causation of the disorder, they may have important effects on its course, as is true of any disorder, organic or functional.

Follow-up research on "borderline psychosis" as a separate group seems to be practically nonexistent. Although Geleerd (1958), Knight (1953), Ekstein and Wallerstein (1954), and the Group for the Study of Borderline Cases in London (Rosenfeld and Sprince, 1963) have described in detail a group of "borderline" children from their clinical practice, this has become a "waste-basket" term to cover psychoses in children other than the very early onset types of autism and symbiosis. Geleerd added to these two a class of "benign" cases characterized by delay in ego development, disturbances in impulse control, poor social adaptation, pervasive and intense anxiety with a whole array of neurotic-like defenses which are only partially successful in allaying anxiety. The Group for the Study of Borderline Cases stressed deficient object relationship.

Rosenfeld and Sprince (1963) point out that the development of the whole personality depends on the capacity for maintaining object relations. The "borderline" child is unable to internalize the object and when threatened with the necessity for separation-individuation during the oedipal stage, regresses to the oral and anal stages with omnipotence and hostile, ambivalent dependence on the mother appearing as two of the foremost clinical signs. Some authors (e.g., Bender, 1956) describe pseudoneurotic and pseudopsychopathic types of the disorder depending on whether neurotic-like defenses or hostile acting out is the observable syndrome.

A few follow-up studies have included later-onset psychoses as one group in their samples. Havelkova (1968) included "pseudoneurotic forms of psychosis" as one of her categories and placed these children with the mildly and moderately affected preschool-age, psychotic children whom she followed for 4 to 12 years. The outcome for the severely affected group (17, or 24%, of her total sample of 71 children) was extremely poor. Of the 54 children in "mild" and "moderate" groups, however, some 35 had moved from an autistic phase through a symbiotic phase to pseudoneurosis by the time of follow-up and another four retained their pseudoneurotic status. Of these "changed" children (i.e., loss of autistic features), 15 were in normal classes, 17 in "opportunity" classes, and 3 had to remain at home.

Havelkova compared a subgroup of children (42) who were treated with a control group (29) of untreated children and found that treatment was unrelated to "emotional" improvement but was related to the child's ability to attend school. Sixty-six percent of the treated and only 17% of the untreated children were in normal schools at follow-up.

Havelkova, like many other researchers in childhood psychosis, points up the central importance of intelligence and warns against diagnostic overoptimism about intellectual "potential." In general, IQ had deteriorated at follow-up for her total group with the largest drop in the group originally described as "mildly disturbed." At follow-up, 44% of the 25 children in this group had IQ's under 70 whereas only one child had been judged originally to have such a low IQ.

In a follow-up of 84 children classified into 7 subtypes of psychosis, Etemad and Szurek (1973) found that the outcome for borderline and "episodic" (acute, late onset) children was significantly better than that of the sample as a whole, while the outcome for the "core" group (infantile autism) was significantly worse than that of the total sample. Even so, only 41% of the borderline patients achieved a "best" rating five years or more after initial diagnosis and to earn this rating the patient had only to have had no further hospitalization and to have achieved independence in one area of life functioning from among employment, marriage, military service, or schooling appropriate to age.

Menolascino and Eaton (1968) included 5 children with a diagnosis of "childhood schizophrenia" in their follow-up of 29 psychotic children who had been originally suspected of being mentally retarded at age 4 years 8 months. At follow-up five years later, of the 5, 3 were in state hospitals and the other two had to be kept at home. These five children had deteriorated in IQ. It is difficult, from the report, to ascertain if these children could be called "borderline" but they were not included in the two other groups: early infantile autism and chronic brain syndrome with psychosis.

The factor of age at onset has received increasing attention as research in the area of psychoses progresses. Acting on Kanner's and Potter's suggestions that young children cannot be expected, because of their primitive state of ego development, to display clinical features with the same degree of elaboration and complexity as found in the adult, Kolvin and his group (1971) in England have carried on a series of studies designed specifically to differentiate psychosis with onset before 3 years of age and characterized by self-isolation from psychosis with onset from 5 to 15 years of age characterized by symptoms of adult schizophrenia, especially hallucinations, delusions, and other thought disorders. Using a sample of 33 late onset and 47 early onset children, they compared the two groups in symptomatology, family and social background, parental personalities, cerebral dysfunction, and cognitive factors. Their findings are summarized here:

1. *Clinically,* the early onset group was characterized by speech anomalies, unusual responses to noises, indifference to pain, stereotyped movements, self-directed aggression, a spread of compulsive acts, and poor relationships with others especially as shown by gaze-avoidance. The late onset group displayed disorders of thought, commonly hallucinated, and showed perplexity or an attitude of suffering.

2. *Family background* differences were found in that more of the early onset children's parents were in the two upper classes and had a lower rate of schizophrenia; there was a trend for first born children in this group to be at great risk. The parents of late onset children were more likely to be in lower classes socially, had a significantly higher rate of schizophrenia, and there was a trend for mothers to be more socially isolated. Testing with the Maudsley Personality Inventory found mothers of the late onset group to be more introverted.

3. *Cerebral dysfunction* was judged to be present in one fourth of the early onset children and low voltage EEG's were much commoner in this group; 46% of this group and 69% of the late onset group showed *no* evidence of cerebral dysfunction.

4. *Intellectual deficit* was severe in the early onset group with only 21% of them testing above 70. In the late onset group, 87% were above this "educationally crucial" cutoff mark. Low IQ tended to be associated

with evidence of cerebral dysfunction in the early onset group and with delayed milestones in the late onset group.

Even when the research sample is adolescents and young adults, the factor of age at onset is apparently important. Pollack et al. (1968) followed a group of 81 "well-educated" and "voluntary" schizophrenic patients three years after their discharge from a hospital where they had been intensively treated with psychotherapy and drugs. The group was divided into adolescents (15-19 years), young adults (20-29 years), and older adults (30-57 years). At followup, the adolescents and young adults had a much poorer outcome on 5 of the 7 variables used and on a global measure of outcome. The variables related to poor outcome were young age at first psychiatric contact, young age at first admission to hospital, relatively low IQ, low socioeconomic status, and two types of childhood diagnosis (asociality and fearful-paranoid).

In summary, there is increasing evidence from research that the psychoses of childhood fall into at least two classes on the issue of their continuity into adulthood. Infantile and symbiotic psychoses do continue as serious disorders into adulthood with improvement in only a small percentage of cases. These disorders do not seem to be of the same nature as adult schizophrenia. Within these early onset groups a distinction must be made on the basis of mutism and/or organic bases as to prognosis. The adult course of the most severely affected infantile psychotic group seems to be a gradual lessening of the autism itself (physical isolation) and of hyperactivity (when present early), a move toward social interaction but with continuing poor peer relationships, and a change in the nature of ritualistic behaviors. Where speech has not been in evidence before 5 years of age, it almost never develops later. Intelligence in this group is not likely to increase but to deteriorate. Schooling seems to hold some slight hope for improvement whereas therapy has not shown promise.

Little research has been done on later onset psychoses. The few studies done suggest that the syndrome is quite different from infantile psychosis and the prognosis somewhat brighter. Borderline psychotic children may cross "the border" into either severe neurosis, usually of an obsessive-compulsive nature, or into psychosis, often of a paranoid type.

Few children with any kind of childhood psychosis have been judged to have "good" adjustment in adulthood. The proportion of neurotic children who attain a good adjustment in adulthood, about two-thirds, is high in comparison to that of psychotic children, which has been estimated from the various studies to be 5 to 17% with only one study reporting a 29% figure. Moreover, the meaning of the "good adjustment" rating for neurotic outcome is quite different from that for the psychotic outcome. In the former case, it usually means adequate social, educational, and occupational functioning while for psychotics it usually means only the ability to function independently.

RESEARCH ON DEVIANT BEHAVIOR AS RELATED TO THE STUDY OF NORMATIVE GROUPS

Longitudinal Studies

The term "longitudinal study" is usually used to refer to repeated observations on the same group of subjects over a long period of time. In 1964, Jerome Kagan (1964) reviewed ten longitudinal research projects which had been initiated in the United States since 1920. They are, with their start-up dates: 1) the Study of the Gifted Child, Stanford University, 1920; 2) Child Research Council Study in Human Development, University of Colorado School of Medicine, 1923; 3) Child to Adult Study, Institute of Child Development at the University of Minnesota, 1925; 4-6) three studies at the University of California Institute of Human Development: the Berkeley Growth Study (1928), the Guidance Study (1928), and the Oakland Growth Study (1931); 7) the Study of Human Development, Fels Research Institute, 1929; 8) the Longitudinal Study of Child Health and Development, Harvard School of Public Health, 1929; 9) the Infancy Coping and Mental Health Studies, the Menninger Foundation, 1948; and 10) Study of Behavioral Development of the New York University School of Medicine, 1956.

These ten projects and a few others in the United States and abroad have all sought, through observation of the same individuals at successive points in time, to trace the incidence, permanence, and change in certain human characteristics over time, but they vary greatly in 1) the ages of the research subjects covered; 2) the comprehensiveness of the subject sample and of the characteristics studied; 3) the regularity with which the observations are made; 4) the techniques of assessment employed, and 5) the level, behavioral versus interpretive, at which judgments are made.

Most of the long-term longitudinal projects were set up originally to provide normative, developmental data in various areas of functioning such as sensory-motor, language, and concept-formation, and in personality characteristics such as aggressiveness, achievement, dependency, dominance, competitiveness, conformity, sociability, and self-role identification. Some of the studies such as the Fels project (Baldwin et al., 1949; Crandall, 1972) and the Berkeley Growth Study (Hunt and Eichorn, 1972) also included assessment of parental behaviors and attitudes and of parent-child inter-action. The methods used cover virtually all those available to the behavioral sciences: psychometrics, projective tests, observation of behavior in the natural setting and in the laboratory, interviews, teachers' ratings, and experimental procedures of various kinds.

The longitudinal studies were concerned, primarily, with tracing "normal" development over long periods of time. There was, at first, little attention paid to symptoms or behavior deviance as such and variables were usually described in terms of central tendencies for each age level. Of course, only a small percentage of the subjects, which usually numbered a few hundred per project, displayed serious behavioral deviance.

The presence of these deviant subjects caught the attention of the researchers, especially when, as in the case of Thomas and Chess (1968), they felt an obligation to offer therapy to those children in whom they had detected disturbance. In addition, clinical researchers interested in the natural history of children's behavior disorders and their continuity into adulthood became aware of the wealth of data available in these longitudinal projects and began to do substudies within them. Their reports describe the incidence of various kinds of deviant characteristics and behaviors at each age level, the consistency and changes in the symptom patterns within the same children over time and, more recently, the relationship of the childhood indices of various kinds to adult adjustment and pathology.

In the last decade or two, there have been several efforts to bring back adults who were, as children, participants in longitudinal projects, to assess their adult adjustment and to relate it to childhood data recorded for them at various age levels. Sometimes the old childhood data had to be recast in terms of personality dimensions that could be compared to current, more clinical assessment of pathology (e.g., Haan, 1972; Livson and Peskin, 1967). In other projects, the data were simply left in original form and, in these (e.g., Hunt and Eichorn, 1972), pathology is simply related to broad personality dimensions of childhood such as "sociability," "achievement orientation," "responsiveness to humor," "passivity," and "cooperativeness" rather than to the more problem-oriented childhood variables such as those used in high risk designs like child guidance follow-up and follow-back studies. The longitudinal study shares with the follow-up and follow-back studies the advantage of having data actually *recorded* during childhood but, in the case of the older, formal longitudinal projects, the variables, as recorded, were often more numerous and less pathology oriented than in clinic populations.

Longitudinal projects also provide consistent data for studying personality development through tracing changes in incidence of different behaviors and characteristics over successive stages within the *group* constituting the project sample as well as in individuals. However, using the *same* individuals for repeated assessment has brought different results as to consistency and change over time than those obtained from cross-sectional studies where the group of subjects is different for each age level.

Gersten and her co-workers (1976) subjected their data on a Manhattan sample of 732 children and adolescents to both cross-sectional and longitudinal analysis. Originally interviewed when their children were 6 to 18 years of age, the mothers were interviewed again some five years later and their responses were recorded about some 287 items of child behavior.

From these items, 12 factors were finally extracted and factor scores were derived for each child at points I and II in time. Neither the results of cross-sectional analysis of factor scores by age levels at Time I nor of that at Time II agreed with the results of the *longitudinal* analysis of mean changes with aging of the same children between the two assessments. Moreover, cross-sectional analysis of factor scores at Time I was not congruent with a cross-sectional analysis of these factors at Time II. In other words, the conclusions as to changes in disturbances with age or developmental trends were quite different according to which type of analysis was conducted. "When the conclusions as to developmental trends as drawn from the Time I cross-sectional analyses and the longitudinal analyses on the set of 12 factors were compared, 42% of those conclusions disagreed" (Gersten et al., p. 123).

The authors point out that change information denotes how the amount of a particular kind of disturbance shown by a *group* of children shifts over time while *stability* information indicates the extent to which *individual* children preserve their rank-ordering within the group. Cross-sectional designs are not suited to trace the developmental course of disturbance within individuals. They do present a picture of the incidence of various problems and characteristics which can serve as a normative background against which to judge how usual or unusual a certain child's behavior is for a particular age.

In addition to providing information as to the incidence of problem behaviors in nonclinical samples, the longitudinal studies have pointed up the importance of age and sex in the incidence of problem behavior and personality characteristics as they relate to personality development and behavior disturbances.

In the California Guidance Study under the direction of Jean Walker Macfarlane (1954), behavioral characteristics of a sizable group of control[1] ("normal") children aged 21 months to 14 years were recorded from mothers' reports at successive age levels and separately for boys and girls, for firstborn and non-firstborn children. Analyses were done on age trends, sex differences, birth order differences; on persistence of and interrelationship among problems; and on relationship of problems to a few other variables such as IQ and personality characteristics in the mother.

This kind of careful and long-lived investigation allows for a detailed account of the changes with age of many characteristics considered to be important to adjustment; it suffers from the progressive loss in the number of children being studied at each successive age. The study started with 116 "control" children at 21 months of age, of which only 41 were still available at age 14 years.

Macfarlane and her group concluded that most problems do not persist

---

[1]"Control" designates subjects of the total sample who were less intensively studied than the project's "guidance group" and who were not offered treatment.

over a long age span and even for short periods of time. They point up five varieties of problems in terms of frequencies at successive age levels, problems that: decline with age; increase with age; reach a peak and subside; decline from a high frequency and then rise again; or show little or no relationship to age. Only three problems proved to be predictive from the 5 and 7 year levels to the 14 year level: overdependence, somberness, and irritability. Macfarlane's group ended their book-length report of this research with a tribute to the "adaptive capacity of the human organism" who uses such a "variety of coping devices" for his "complex set of tasks."

Incidence of Problems in "Normal" Samples

When cross-sectional and longitudinal data have been utilized as "norms" against which to evaluate the incidence rates of problem behaviors in children referred to clinics, it has become apparent that many of the problems that are the bases of referral are "normal" at certain age levels. Leo Kanner (1960) raised this issue after hearing the results of an epidemiological survey of behavior characteristics of public school children conducted in Buffalo a few years earlier (Lapouse and Monk, 1958). These authors point out that the high incidence of problems such as fears and worries (43%), overactivity (49%), and loss of temper (80% at a once-a-month rate) among their 6-12 year old sample raises the question of whether these problems can be considered to be indicative of psychiatric disorder or whether they are, instead, "transient developmental phenomena in essentially normal children" (Kanner, 1960, p. 19).

   Estimates of the number of grade school children who are maladjusted to a degree requiring clinical help have varied depending on many different group characteristics of the children, on who does the assessment of disturbance, and on the definition of maladjustment. Teachers' reports include Wickman's (1928) widely quoted figure of 7% of elementary school children with serious behavior problems, Rogers' (1942) 12% figure where teachers' judgment was one of several criteria, and Ullman's (1952b) 8% figure for ninth grade children considered "likely sooner or later to have serious problems of adjustment and to need special help or care because of such problems" (p. 1221). Glidewell et al. (1959) confined their survey to third grade pupils in St. Louis County. Using Ullman's scale of adjustment, teachers placed 28% of their 830 children in the "subclinically" and "clinically disturbed" categories. The latter category contained 68, or 8.2%, of the 830 children, remarkably close to Ullman's 8% of ninth graders with "serious" problems of adjustment.

   In general, when those with "moderate" maladjustment are added to the seriously maladjusted, the figure is likely to be 20 to 35% in a public school sample. The initiation, in 1958, of a Mental Health Project in the Monroe County, New York, public schools to detect early school malfunctioning and the existence of a cumulative psychiatric register in the same county allowed Emory Cowen (1973) and his research group to 1) assess the incidence of "moderate to severe" maladaptation in the firt three grades and 2) to trace most of these children some 11 to 13 years later through the Psychiatric Register for evidence of psychiatric referral and service data. About one third of the children were "tagged" in first and/or third grade as "vulnerable" on the basis of ineffective school performance and behavior. Multiple data were available on which to base the clinical prognostic judgment of "red tag" or not "red tag." They included social work interviews with mothers, achievement scores, psychological evaluation, classroom observations of the children and teachers' reports.

It was found that first-grade red-tag children were doing significantly less well than the nonred-tag children on a variety of behavioral and educational indices both at the end of their third grade and throughout their entire elementary school years. Some 487 children, all of whom had been part of a preventive mental health program, were considered in the follow-up. Of these, 50 individuals (or nearly 10%) were found in the Psychiatric Register and a disproportionately high percentage of them (68%) had been screened as vulnerable (tagged red) in the first three grades as compared to the base-rate frequency of one in three red-tags in the primary grades.

This research lends credence to the possibility of early detection, in school settings, of later maladjustments even though it does not give much support to the long-term value of a preventive program of the limited kind then being offered in the Primary Mental Health Project. Interesting also, sociometric ratings by 8- and 9-year-old peers best predicted later psychiatric difficulty This finding agrees with those of several other investigators (Mednick and Schulsinger, 1970; Roff, 1974; Ullman, 1952b) that status among and relationship to peers are important variables in later adjustment.

One of the most careful studies comparing children referred to child guidance clinics with a control group from the same large sample of public school children who had never attended such a clinic was done in the early 1960s by Sheperd, Oppenheim, and Mitchell in Buckinghamshire County in England (1966). Both groups were drawn from an original sample of 6920 children who represented 1 in 10 children between 5 and 15 years of age attending "local authority" schools in the County in 1961. The survey yielded a high (over 90%) rate of response to questionnaires about the children sent to parents and teachers.

For the comparison study itself, 50 children attending child guidance clinics for the first time in 1962 were matched with 50 nonclinic school children for age, sex, and behavior similar to the clinic children. In order to have a clinic sample most comparable in behavioral characteristics to the general school sample, all clinic referrals with psychotic, serious behavior disorders, and/or organic diagnoses were excluded as well as those forced by the court to attend the clinics and those in residential schools or children's homes. Also excluded from the clinic sample were children under age 5 and over 15. The 50 children finally selected represented about 3 out of the 4 children of school age consecutively chosen as they came to the clinic for a diagnostic interview.

Mothers of the experimental and control groups were interviewed. Their responses to the survey questionnaire and, additionally, in the case of the clinic children, their reasons for bringing their child to the clinic served as a basis for the interviews. Much other information was obtained for both groups of children including family background factors, parents' marital and emotional status, the attitudes and reactions of family members and of others to the child's behavior , and the actions taken to deal with it.

When all 100 children were rated "blindly" by five clinicians on a 5-point scale of disturbance from very mild (1) to very severe (5) there was only a nonsignificant trend toward more severe ratings for the clinic children. Among the 50 matched pairs, the averaged ratings were *identical* for 27 pairs and less than one point apart in an additional 11 pairs. In 75% of the pairs, the *same* ratings were given to both children by at least one rater. Although the authors claim that this comparison is convincing evidence that children who are referred to clinics may show little difference in degree of disturbance from other children of like age, sex, and behavioral characteristics drawn from the same source, it must be remembered that the most disturbed children in the clinic group had been excluded from the sample.

One factor that did distinguish the two groups was the mother's reaction to the child's behavior. Significantly, more clinic mothers than controls felt bewildered, unable to cope, or worried about their child's future welfare or present unhappiness. In light of the small difference in the severity of disturbance between the clinic and control groups, it may be that children often get to clinics because of the parents' tendency to worry or lose confidence in their ability to cope with their children's problems. This hypothesis gains some support from another finding, that is, more clinic mothers saw themselves as "suffering from nerves" than did nonclinic mothers. Moreover, 10 of the clinic children had suffered the loss of one parent permanently, compared with 3 in the nonclinic group.

These two groups of children were reassessed through parental interviews two years later (1964). Of the original 100 sets of parents, 87 were available and willing to cooperate. The interviewers were provided the old data and ratings on the children but references as to which children had attended clinics and/or had received treatment were omitted. At the second assessment of the children, 55, or 63% had improved over the interim period, 12 (24%) had remained the same, and only 11 (13%) had deteriorated. There was no significant difference, moreover, between clinic and nonclinic children in these change data. Among the clinic children, outcome was not related to number of treatment sessions or to initial disturbance. The authors conclude that "on

the basis of the study, then, we would suggest that many so-called disturbances of behavior are no more than temporary exaggerations of widely-
distributed reaction-patterns. The transient nature of these reactions is
demonstrated by the tendency to spontaneous improvement in the untreated
children...." (p. 47). Sheperd et al.'s results warrant this conclusion in so far
as the limitations of his study allow. This group excluded clinic children with
severe disturbances, and behaviors of children were judged only from parental
reports.

The proportion of children in longitudinal studies who are found, in the
course of assessment on many personality or behavioral characteristics, to
have "problems" is often much higher than in the school surveys. For
example, Thomas and Chess (1976) found that 48 of the 136 children they
followed from early infancy into adolescence presented symptoms qualifying
them for psychiatric evaluation and almost half of these 48 did so between
ages 3 and 5 years. This study demonstrates the high yield of disturbance
when clinicians do the assessment and when "symptoms" are the basis for
their judgment. In the Thomas and Chess group, half of the "disturbed"
children had "improved" or "recovered" before adolescence. The authors
themselves are aware of the broad scope of their definition of disturbance.
They referred for psychiatric evaluation children with even mild behavior
problems and they state that many "would have recovered spontaneously and
not come to psychiatric attention if they had not been subjects in the longitudinal study" (p. 540).

The percentage of "disturbed children" in a general school sample who are
referred for help is, of course, very small. Sheperd et al. (1966, p. 47) quote a
general practitioner as estimating that for each child referred to child guidance clinics there are 5, equally disturbed, who are not referred.

Follow-up of Longitudinal Study Subjects

Several recent projects have made use of the copious childhood data of
longitudinal studies to determine the consistency of personality characteristics over time and their individual capacity to predict outcomes later in time,
especially from childhood stages to adulthood. The Institute of Human
Development at Berkeley has succeeded in following up and interviewing
some 171 subjects as adults who were part of the Oakland Growth Study
(OGS) and the Guidance Study (GS) in childhood and adolescence (Haan,
1972). The Guidance Study subjects averaged 30 years of age and the Oakland
Growth subjects 37 at the first follow-up, 1957-60. They were interviewed
again about ten years later, 1969-72.

One of the earlier reports of these longitudinal follow-up projects is that of
Livson and Peskin (1967). They used a sample of 31 men and 31 women at an

average age of 31 years who had complete childhood data from the Guidance Study at four periods of life: 5-7 years, 8-10 years, 11-13 years, and 14-16 years. The data were based on direct observations, child interviews, and teachers' ratings. Item-cluster analyses of the data yielded 24 clusters for boys and 26 for girls with 5 to 7 repeatable clusters at any given age period. Cluster scores were computed for each subject.

These 62 subjects were interviewed intensively in adulthood and interview data were recorded for the 100 items of the California Q sort. This method of personality analysis describes ideal psychological health in terms of characteristics such as dependability, responsibility, warmth, compassion, givingness, productivity, awareness of and insight into one's own behavior and motives, ethical behavior, and interest in members of the opposite sex. It excludes a rating of psychopathology as such and describes the *unhealthy* adult as one who has a brittle ego-defense system, becomes disorganized under stress, feels cheated by life, gives up and withdraws, is deceitful, distrustful, self-defeating, anxious, and fearful.

Each adult's health score was determined by correlating actual Q-sort with that of the "ideal" health Q-sort as determined by the consensus of several experienced clinicians. When the item scores for the 4 stages of childhood were related to the subjects' adult psychological health score, Livson and Peskin found that at only one childhood stage, that of preadolescence, age 11-13 years, were the scores predictive to health in adulthood and that the predictors were different for boys and girls.

The overall correlation for the 62 subjects from preadolescence to adulthood was .58. The predictive variables for boys were "relatively extroverted, expressive, immune to irritability and temper tantrums" and for girls: "relatively independent, a confident, inquiring orientation, hearty attitude toward food" (pp. 514-515). The other three age periods yielded correlations of only .03 to .36 with adolescence the least predictive stage of all (r =.03). Moreover, a *total* problem score of the 4 stages did not correlate significantly to adult health assessment.

These authors interpret their findings in psychoanalytic terms and suggest that the importance of the 11 to 13 year period in childhood may be because this is the age of "responsiveness to and mastery of social reality" (p. 515). They refer to Helene Deutsch and Harry Sullivan as agreeing essentially with this view in contrast to others like Erikson who stresses, instead, the importance of adolescence. Interestingly, the picture of the potentially unhealthy boy that Livson draws is remarkably like the ambivert of the Dallas study (Michael et al., 1957), socially withdrawn and aloof but having little control over hostility (temper, irritability, explosiveness).

Impressed by these unexpected results, the authors pursued the analysis of their data along other lines (Peskin and Livson, 1972). When they looked at the childhood data of one group of subjects who had high scores on psychological health as adults in spite of relatively poor scores in preadolescent behaviors, they found that the boys in this group came from emotionally stable and relatively happy families and that they had a closer relationship to their fathers at ages 21 months to 3 years than did those whose adult status was correctly predicted from their preadolescent behavior. For the girls of this subsample, their greater closeness to mother in early life was the differentiating feature. Peskin and Livson point to these results as demonstrating the possibility that there are *alternative* routes to adult psychological health, in this case, early family determinants *or* positive preadolescent behaviors.

Another reexamination of earlier data (Peskin, 1972) was concerned with the failure of the adolescent period (ages 14 to 16) to predict to adulthood. When Peskin assessed the predictive power of each specific behavior from their preadolescent and adolescent values together, he found that the *only* adolescent behavior that forecast adult health did so in a direction *opposite* from their preadolescent effects. For both sexes, *no* adolescent effect emerged except as a reversal of a corresponding preadolescent effect. The patterns were quite different for boys and girls, however. Highest psychological health in adulthood in boys is related to a reversal from placidity and stolidness in preadolescence to irritability in adolescence; for healthy female adulthood, the sequence is from independence and self-confidence in preadolescence to dependence and low self-confidence in adolescence.

Continuity of personality has also been studied in tracing *patterns* of traits. A second project using the Oakland Growth and Guidance Study subjects and reported by Norma Hann (1972) developed "typologies" of personality from combining Q-sort data based on adult interviews and similar Q-sort items based on the various kinds of data from childhood. Five male and 6 female types were identified by Q-factoring of these data. The 11 types showed differing degrees of continuity from junior high school age through senior high school to adulthood.

One typology in males and one in females were "substantially"continuous in traits over this 20- to 25-year period. Both these groups, the male "Ego Resilients" and the "Female Prototypes" are described in positive terms such as poised, intellectual, well-socialized, comfortable with peers, parents, and other adults. They were the largest of the groups in the sample, together accounting for 38 subjects (28%) of the 134 subjects who could be cast into types. This finding lends support to findings in other research that psychological health in childhood is more predictive to similar adult status than is ill health.

The 9 other types displayed varying degrees of continuity and of eventual adjustment. Some displayed initial and continuing maladjustment; other types, especially male "Belated Adjusters" and female "Cognitive Copers" improved dramatically in adulthood while 2 other types were marked by deterioration from junior high school to adulthood and substantial discontinuity.

Important findings in relation to the question of whether disturbance continues into adulthood are that *no* pathognomonic traits *consistently* characterized the early adolescents who became troubled later and that the female type who dropped markedly in adjustment (Hyper-feminine Regressive) was quite different from the male type showing the greatest drop (the Anomic Extroverts). When specific variables rather than typology were examined, few of the variables showed great continuity *even* for those subjects who changed least in the overall sense. Exceptions included speed and restiveness of reaction for both sexes and, for men, pathological indices evidenced in passivity, resignation, and uncertainty. Female continuity of traits was *very* sparse in this period from young adolescence to adulthood.

Anna Freud (1958a) referred to this phenomenon of adolescent change. She held that 1) normal adolescence is by its nature an interruption of peaceful growth, and 2) that the upholding of a steady equilibrium during the adolescent period is in itself abnormal (p. 275). The normal adolescent deals with the anxieties engendered by the quantitative and qualitative increase in drives by flight from his infantile objects, by displacement of libido onto parent substitutes, and by *defenses* which often appear as behavioral *opposites* of the individual's previous behaviors such as denial of positive feelings and reaction formations in which positive feelings are turned into rebellion and contempt toward parents and independence may temporarily revert to childish dependence. These defenses are used until drive activity can be reintegrated into the more mature personality. They are consistent with the reversals of the Peskin and Livson research.

Anna Freud also drew attention to a picture of true pathology in adolescence, one in which the danger of being overwhelmed by the id is so great and resulting anxiety so intense that "total war is waged against the pursuit of pleasure as such" (p. 274). When this rigidity persists, serious pathology is seen in adulthood. This picture seems to be similar to the "Vulnerable Overcontrollers" among Haan's types who presented a continuous picture of maladjustment from junior high school through young adulthood.

These results point out the complexity of relating childhood variables to adult outcome with the sex of the child and the age from which predictions are made representing only two, and perhaps the least complex, considerations. The findings suggest also that follow-up research confined to one sex or to one age period of childhood may yield results which show childhood is predictive or nonpredictive depending on whether the researcher did or did not happen to pick the "right" sex or age period. Where the two sexes are combined, effects for some variables may cancel each other out. More impressive than their importance in presenting possible reasons for conflicting research results, moreover, is the contribution of the longitudinal studies to the understanding of personality development. Personality progresses from infancy to adulthood in a series of transformations which are often observable at one period of time as behaviors that reverse those observed in preceding or other earlier periods. In adolescence, the appearance of less healthy behaviors in a previously well-adjusted child may be a frequent prelude to adult psychological health.

RESEARCH CONCERNED WITH CHILD THERAPY OUTCOME

This comprehensive, although not exhaustive, review of child psychotherapy outcome studies focuses on the following questions: 1) Is child psychotherapy effective? 2) For which children—diagnostic group, age, sex, symptomatology—is psychotherapy effective? 3) Are specific therapy conditions such as theoretical approach, length of therapy, skill of therapist, and type of therapy related to outcome?

An underlying assumption in most programs of child therapy is that treatment of parents is an essential component of child therapy, yet most outcome studies reported to date do not assess parental response to therapy. Parental involvement or lack of involvement in therapy as well as parental pathology is addressed in some of them, but change or outcome of work with parents and the adequacy of parental adjustment or functioning at follow-up was not assessed in the studies reviewed. (One exception was noted in a study by Lessing and Schilling [1966] which assessed mothers at point of closing.) The failure to consider parental change constitutes a serious limitation in child therapy outcome research, if the generally accepted belief in the effect of parental influences on child development is valid.

Effectiveness of Psychotherapy

Two authors have presented comprehensive reviews of child psychotherapy or casework outcome studies: Levitt (1957, 1963, 1971) and Fischer (1976).

Levitt's first review (1957) included 18 studies, and all but one of them reported outcome both at closing and at follow-up. In this review he included only studies that evaluated neurotic children, although he indicates a few children exhibiting delinquent behavior may have been included. His second review (1963) included 22 studies of neurotic, psychotic, and acting out children. Over half of these studies evaluated outcome at follow-up rather than at closing.

In the third review (1971), Levitt included data from his previous reviews. He aggregated the results of 47 studies of therapy outcome. Neurotic, psychotic, and acting out children, a total of 5140 children, were assessed at closing; 66.4% of them were rated improved. In addition, he reported follow-up outcome data for those children who were diagnosed neurotic (4219) but did not include those diagnosed as psychotic or acting out in the follow-up assessment. Of the neurotic children, 78.2% were rated improved at follow-up. The time interval between closing and follow-up varied considerably with an estimated median interval of 4.8 years.

The reason why psychotic and acting out children were eliminated from the report of follow-up data is not clear, but may be related to the absence of follow-up data for these groups as well as the limited number of children (601, or 11%) in these diagnostic categories. The higher proportion of children rated as improved at *follow-up* as contrasted with the ratings at closing may be partly related to the elimination of the psychotic and acting out children from the follow-up data. Since the improvement rate at closing differs somewhat for different diagnostic categories, it is likely that these differences would also be evident at follow-up. The improvement rate for acting out children (55%) at closing is considerably lower than that for neurotic (67.4%) and psychotic (65.1%) children. Nevertheless, some improvement seems to occur over time as indicated by comparing the improvement rates of neurotic chidren at closing (67.4%) and at follow-up (78.2%).

Levitt reports that in studies that utilized control groups, which are most often composed of defectors, that is, those who had completed diagnostic procedures but had not participated in therapy, the improvement rate was about the same in treated and untreated groups. Levitt suggested that the analysis of outcome studies challenged many of the procedures traditionally followed by child guidance clinics and he proposed that prognostic criteria and treatment procedures be reconsidered.

Fischer (1976), in reviewing 17 studies of casework, concluded that these studies showed that treatment was ineffective or harmful. Fischer included studies in which individualized service was provided by a caseworker and in which there was an untreated control group or a control group treated by nonprofessionals. Of the 17 studies reviewed by Fischer, 10 were focused on treatment of children. Of these 10 studies, one by Lehrman et al. (1949) claimed positive results from treatment, but Fischer challenged the interpretation of the data in that study. Seven of the 10 studies were of delinquency prevention or control programs; such programs have generally shown rather poor results.

Fischer's (1976) review and conclusions were discussed by different writers in his book, *The Effectiveness of Social Casework*. Several writers disagreed with Fischer's conclusions and suggested that the studies reviewed were not adequate to support or negate the effectiveness of casework.

These two reviews point to the lack of evidence to support the belief that psychotherapy is effective in helping children and in reducing adult pathology. However, a number of serious methodological issues are evident in trying to assess psychotherapy outcome.

Assessment of Outcome. First, how are the effects or outcome of psychotherapy evaluated? Strupp and Hadley (1977) propose a tripartite model for evaluating mental health and psychotherapy outcome. This model was derived from examination of the values of society, the individual, and the mental health professional. To assess therapy outcome, they suggested that three dimensions of a person's functioning be considered: adaptive behavior, sense of well-being, and personality structure.

Child therapy outcome research has tended to assess outcome on the basis of behavioral change or adjustment or on the basis of personality structure. Only one of the studies reviewed, Leventhal and Weinberger (1975), considered the individual's sense of well-being. In this study of brief treatment, mother and father were each asked at closing and at follow-up, one and a half years later, if therapy had helped each of them and their child and how each of them was doing. Ratings of helpfulness and of adjustment were derived by combining the responses of each parent in regard to self-assessment and his or her assessment of the other parent and the child. At closing, 85 to 90% of the parents reported that each of them and their child were doing a little better or much better. At follow-up, parents' sense of how each of them and their child were doing declined slightly; 66% of the fathers, 83% of the mothers, and 89% of the children were doing a little or much better according to the combined parental reports.

The same process of combining parental responses to the question about helpfulness of treatment was utilized. At closing 85 to 93% of the parents reported that therapy had helped each of them and their child a little or a great deal. At follow-up, according to parental reports, therapy had helped 85% of the mothers, 69% of the fathers, and 77% of the children a little or a great deal.

Therapists also rated improvement at closing, but their ratings were less positive than the combined parent ratings. Therapists rated changes in pathology based on the difference in degree of pathology as rated after the first interview and at closing. In brief therapy 66% of the children showed positive change, slightly less than half the mothers, and 36% of the fathers. However, it was noted that parents were rated as being less pathological than children initially, so there was less opportunity for positive change.

Although only this study touched on well-being, it relied on parental reports and did not directly assess the child's well-being. Also, the follow-up data were obtained by mailed questionnaire and the response rate was low.

Studies (Goldfarb, 1970; Waldron, 1976; Weiss and Burke, 1970) which included some sort of assessment of personality structure at *follow-up* tended to show less positive outcomes than the generally expected rate of positive outcome, 78.2%, reported in Levitt's review.

Goldfarb (1970) followed up a group of 46 schizophrenic children of mean ages 7 years when treated and 16.8 years at follow-up. He utilized an ego status scale which assessed impairment in ego functioning and social adjustment.

Two levels of impairment of ego functioning and social adjustment were utilized at follow-up: 1) *Grossly impaired ego functioning* was "characterized by extremely disordered psychotic behavior and at times apparent mental retardation." Capacity for self-care was totally lacking or deficient. 2) *Mildly impaired to normal ego functioning* was "characterized by adaptive capacity, educational response, and social behavior sufficient to enable the child to attend school and to live in the community."

At follow-up 33% of the subjects were rated mildly impaired to normal in ego functioning and 67% were rated grossly impaired in ego functioning. The grossly impaired group manifested psychotic patterns of adjustment. At follow-up 50% of the subjects were institutionalized. The relatively poor outcome of these subjects, in contrast to Levitt's reviews, is probably related to the severity of disturbance in childhood. Goldfarb's subjects manifested severe childhood impairment which necessitated residential treatment while Levitt reported follow-up data on outpatient, neurotic subjects.

In contrast to Goldfarb's study, Waldron (1976) followed up a less disturbed group of 42 children, those with a childhood diagnosis of neurosis. Follow-up at mean age 22 years included a clinical interview which utilized the CAPPS and a Health Sickness Rating Scale (HSR). Of those subjects, 40%, or 17, were given psychiatric diagnoses, while 60% did not receive diagnoses on the CAPPS, an instrument designed to produce reliable and valid psychiatric diagnoses through analysis of various scales of symptomatology, adjustment, and functioning.

On the HSR scale, 76% of the subjects were rated mildly, moderately, or severely ill, while 24% were rated as healthy or minimally ill. Thus three fourths of the subjects were rated as having mildly to severely impaired mental health at follow-up, but only two fifths of them had sufficient impairment to warrant a psychiatric diagnosis. This difference between the proportion of subjects given psychiatric diagnoses and ratings of impaired mental health can be attributed primarily to the category of mild impairment. Only 2 of 13 subjects in this category were given psychiatric diagnoses.

A comparison of these former clinic patients and a control group showed the childhood neurotics to be significantly more disturbed at follow-up than the controls who were selected from the subjects' childhood school classmates. None of the controls received a specific diagnosis on the CAPPS program, and only 15% of the controls were rated mildly or moderately ill on the HSR. Differences in the two groups were especially pronounced in the area of interpersonal relationships with 79% of the former patients and 25% of the controls showing more than minimal impairment in this area.

A third study, that of Weiss and Burke (1970), reported impressions of the differences evident in assessing adaptation and mental status. They followed up 14 school phobic children at ages 18 to 26, and reported that their adaptation was generally good, although all but one had neurotic or personality problems.

There is considerable variation in the focus of assessments of therapy effects. Some studies focused on change or improvement in the child while others focused on the adequacy or healthiness of his functioning or adjustment. Is therapy effective if the child shows some improvement but still exhibits some impairment, or is therapy effective only if adequate adjustment or mental health is achieved? In his comparision of a number of studies, Levitt (1957) considered therapy effective if there was improvement or adequate adjustment. He included both outcomes under one heading of improvement.

Individuals listed as "much improved, improved, partially improved, successful, partially successful, adjusted, partially adjusted, satisfactory" etc., will be grouped under the general heading of Improved . . . (p. 189).

Several studies assessed outcome at follow-up by rating improvement (Leventhal and Weinberger, 1975; Levy, 1969; Lo, 1973; Lehrman et al., 1949; Rosenthal and Levine, 1970; Witmer and Keller, 1942). These studies showed a partial or full improvement in 53 to 84% of the children assessed at follow-up. A few studies took into account the relationship of rated success of therapy at closing and at follow-up. Witmer and Keller (1942) reported a follow-up improvement rate of 83% for children considered successfully treated at closing. Of those rated as improved at closing, 48% were rated improved at follow-up.

A few studies which rate adjustment at follow-up in contrast to improvement show lower success rates. However, these differences may be related to the type of children studied; to the seriousness of disturbance in the children of these studies, for example, the psychotic and severely disturbed children of the Davids and Salvatore (1976) and Goldfarb (1970) studies; or to the utilization of clinical assessments which may get at disturbance not evident on a more superficial level.

Time of Outcome Assessment. The time at which therapy is evaluated and the age of the children when followed up seem to influence outcome. Levitt's 1971 review reported improvement rates of 66.4% at closing and 78.2% at follow-up. Thus, further improvement occurred with time. However, of the studies reviewed by Levitt, those in which the assessment was done at follow-up were studies of neurotic children only, whereas those with ratings at close of treatment included neurotic, psychotic, and acting out children. The Levitt review points up the difficulty in comparing studies which differ on important variables.

There is growing evidence that the age of children is an important variable in assessing their functioning or mental health. Longitudinal studies (Thomas and Chess, 1968; Gersten, 1976) emphasize the changing nature of children's behavior and the development or disappearance of symptoms which may occur simply as a part of the developmental process.

Thomas and Chess in their study of temperament identified 42 children with behavior disorders. Of these children, 64% showed improvement one to two years later. Gersten reported that aggressive or conduct disorder types of behavior continue over time or increase, while neurotic types of disturbance tend to be outgrown by mid-adolescence. She suggested that the age at which a child obtains treatment influences outcome. Masterson (1967) followed up disturbed adolescents from ages 16 to 21 and found that 62% continued to show moderate or severe impairment. Witmer and Keller (1942) found that subjects 18 years old or older at follow-up were more likely to be in the improvement category than those younger than 18 years at follow-up. Morris et al. (1956) followed up a group of hospitalized children who were 24 to 35 years of age at follow-up. He stated that most of these children improved in the hospital and for a year after leaving the hospital, then their adjustment fluctuated until age 18. He concluded that assessment at age 18 and beyond provided a more accurate reflection of final outcome than assessment at younger ages.

Shore and Massimo (1973) reported data on 10 subjects who were 15 to 17 years old at time of treatment and 25 to 27 years old at follow-up. Eight of the 10 were adjusting adequately and there had been little change over the 10 year period; those who started doing well in treatment continued and those doing poorly at time of treatment continued to be maladjusted.

Since many of the therapy outcome studies have followed up children who were still in childhood and early adolescence, it seems unlikely that the effects of therapy could be assessed adequately. Heinicke (1969) stresses the necessity of determining the developmental status of a child in order to evaluate treatment. This assessment is necessary both when the child is treated and at follow-up. Some reports do not provide sufficient data to determine the subjects' ages at both time points and others cover a rather wide age range so that the potential variation in therapeutic effects for different age groups could not be assessed.

Control Groups. In attempting to answer the question of the effects of therapy, a number of studies have compared treated (experimental) with nontreated (control) subjects, whereas a few studies have contrasted several types of treatment, primarily brief and long-term. In general, follow-up assessments of experimental and control groups do not show significant differences in improvement rates.

Considerable debate exists regarding the proper choice of a control group.

Most studies have utilized what Levitt calls a "defector" group; children who came to mental health settings, participated in a diagnostic process, but were not seen in therapy. Generally, these children were comparable to the treated groups in areas such as age, sex, diagnosis, family characteristics, and severity of disturbance. Levitt (1957) compared 208 defectors with 132 children who received treatment and found the two groups did not differ signficantly in relation to most of the 61 variables analyzed. Lehrman et al. (1949) and Witmer and Keller (1942) found slight differences in their treatment and defector control groups at time of childhood evaluation. Witmer and Keller reported differences in diagnosis and family environment; Lehrman et al. reported differences in diagnosis in the two groups.

Although evidence both supports and negates the comparability of control and treatment groups, they differ in one major way. Parents of defector children usually chose not to participate in therapy or to have their children involved in treatment. The meaning of this decision is not known. For some families it could reflect a change or improvement in the child and family after referral. It may indicate that parents and child felt they received some help through the diagnostic process. Although parent guidance is not usually included in the diagnostic process, some suggestions and recommendations may be provided to parents and these may lead to changes which preclude the necessity for treatment.

The effectiveness of parent guidance was reported by Thomas et al. (1968) in their longitudinal study in which some children were identified as having behavior disorders. Therapists provided an average of 2.7 sessions to parents in which direct advice and guidance were offered. Fifty percent of the parents responded to this approach and were able to modify their functioning; their children were likely to improve if the parents shifted.

Another possible explanation of the differences between families who choose to follow through with treatment and those who do not may be related to parental anxiety and resistance, neither of which is ordinarily assessed in comparing treatment and control groups. The diagnostic process may serve to heighten anxiety or resistance in some families and to reduce these factors in others. Either an increase or reduction in anxiety could lead families toward or away from treatment, while an increase in resistance would lead to an avoidance of treatment.

Parental Outcome. Historically, child guidance clinics have been the primary providers of child therapy. Until recently the predominant approach to therapy was psychoanalytically oriented and the importance of the parent-child relationship in contributing to pathology or in promoting healthy development was recognized. Consequently, it was expected that one or both parents would be involved in counseling or therapy along with the child. It is surprising, therefore, that so little attention has been given to evaluating parental response to therapy in research attempting to assess the effects of therapy.

Levitt (1971) referred to several studies which related outcome to the person who has the focus of treatment: child only; mother and child; mother and father; mother, father, and child. The findings were inconclusive; however, most of those studies considered only who was the focus of treatment and did not assess the response of the parents to treatment when involved, nor their adjustment at follow-up.

There is some support for the importance of assessing parental functioning and improvement to assess child therapy outcome adequately. As reported previously, Thomas et al. (1968) showed a link between parental change and child behavior. Lehrman (1949) reported that children with two adequate parents responded to therapy more positively than those with one or both parents who were inadequate or psychiatrically disturbed. Goldfarb (1970) in a follow-up study of schizophrenic children discharged from a residential treatment program, provided a clinical impression that children's deterioration after discharge was associated with disturbed families, while improvement after discharge was related to favorable family situations. Lessing and Schilling (1966) examined the relationship between mother's improvement and child's improvement at closing and reported a significant relationship between the two.

Further support for the interdependence of mother and child improvement was provided by Heinicke (1976) in a study of treatment of mothers of preschool children. The children were in day care centers but were not given therapy. Treated parents and their children were compared to children whose parents did not receive treatment. Treated parents changed in a positive direction as people and in their parental functioning. Their children scored higher in IQ and child development ratings than the children whose mothers did not participate in the therapy programs. These differences continued through kindergarten.

Although the interrelationship of parent and child and the influence of parental functioning on child development is theoretically based and has been incorporated in most child therapy practice, it has not been considered in most outcome studies. The few studies described above give support to the assumptions underlying practice. However, these assumptions are now being challenged by some professionals and new treatment approaches are evolving. For example, the usual pattern of requiring the parents to participate if the child is treated may be modified so that only the child is treated or only the parents are treated.

Variables Related to Outcome

Evidence pertaining to identifying the variables which may be related to treatment outcome is minimal. Heinicke and Strassman (1975) questioned much of the outcome research because it is based on the general question of therapy efficacy rather than focused on the conditions in which psychotherapy brings about the enhanced development of the child. Heinicke and Strassman's excellent paper focuses on the methodological issues involved in therapy outcome research, presents a number of suggestions for more effective research, and reviews studies which have examined variables considered to be relevant to outcome. Some of the most important variables are the child's developmental status, kinds of problems, diagnosis, parental impact, and age. In addition, therapeutic variables such as frequency of sessions, duration of treatment, type of treatment, and characteristics of the therapist are considered important but have received minimal attention in child therapy research.

There is some evidence, according to Robins (1972), that in certain types of childhood disorders the prognosis for adult life is poor. Robins' concern was with predicting adult adjustment rather than with treatment outcome. However, if certain types of child disorders seem to lead to adult maladjustment, it may be that treatment will be unsuccessful for these disorders, even though, as Levitt (1971) has indicated, these children may be the ones in greatest need of clinic service. Robins identified childhood psychosis and serious antisocial behavior as having a poor prognosis and neurotic disorders as having a good prognosis for adult adjustment. Some treatment outcome studies of childhood psychosis show a poor response to treatment. Goldfarb (1970) reported 67% of schizophrenics treated at age 7 had severe disturbance at age 16.8 years. Bomberg et al. (1973) reported good outcome for only 28% of the psychotic children they followed up at ages 6 to 17 years. Davids (1972) reported good adjustment for 40% of psychotic or severely disturbed children who were 10 to 28 years old at follow-up.

A few studies have focused on therapeutic variables in assessing outcome. Perhaps most llustrative is Heinicke's (1969) study in which two groups of children were seen with different frequency; one time per week or four times per week for 1½ to 2½ years. The groups did not differ at closing but the more frequently treated subjects showed better ego integration at follow-up 1 and 2 years later than did the less frequently treated subjects.

SUMMARY

Child therapy research has focused on assessment of the effects of therapy. However, the normal developmental processes of childhood, the changes in symptomatic behavior with age, and the influence of parental and other environmental forces on the child increase the complexity of isolating and assessing therapeutic effects. In addition, treatment can be expected to have differential effects according to the type and severity of childhood disturbances. The studies reported have included a wide range of disturbances and this variety contributes further to the difficulty of comparing findings of different studies.

In presenting their tripartite model for evaluating psychotherapy, Strupp and Hadley (1977) raise the issue of the criteria on which to evaluate outcome. There is also wide variation in the length and type of treatment provided, skill and experience of the therapists, and the treatment approaches and techniques utilized, as well as variations in the age of children when treated and at follow-up.

Although the preponderance of the findings question the efficacy of treatment, the complexity of assessing treatment outcome and the methodological problems involved have limited their interpretation and point to the need for long-term follow-up studies, focused on specific aspects of treatment, carried out with homogeneous groups of children, and assessed at outcome through multiple measures of change and adjustment.

CHAPTER 4

The Follow-Up Study

This follow-up study was designed to avoid some of the major deficiencies apparent in the foregoing review of research relating childhood characteristics to adult mental health and to try to shed light on the reasons for conflicting results from those studies. Some research has led to the finding that serious disturbances in adulthood were forecast by certain symptoms and behaviors in children (Bender, 1969; Bronner, 1944; Morris et al., 1956; Robins, 1966; Waldron, 1976). Other studies suggest that many children seen in clinics for evaluation do not, even without treatment, present serious behavior deviance and/or mental illness in adulthood (Morris et al., 1954; Robins, 1966; Roff, 1974). Some limitations of other studies are summarized here.

1. *Limitations in the variety of childhood disturbances included in a study.*

In most studies of "high risk" children, researchers are interested in a particular diagnostic or familial category of childhood such as schizophrenic children (Bender, 1969; Goldfarb, 1970), juvenile delinquents (Jenkins, 1960; Glueck and Glueck, 1940), sociopathic personality (Jenkins, 1960; Morris et al., 1956; Robins, 1966), or children of schizophrenic parents (Anthony, 1968). Even when the sample has been a child guidance group, attention may have been focused primarily on one diagnostic group within that sample, such as the shy, withdrawn children of the Dallas Follow-up Study (Morris et al., 1954).

2. *Insufficent data in the original assessment.*

Since they were usually planned long after the children had been seen for assessment, previous studies have been based on a few but never *all* of the following kinds of dynamic and behavioral assessment procedures: application data, developmental questionnaire, list of symptoms and behavior, extensive social history, psychological test battery, psychiatric interview, and diagnostic conference conclusions.

The Robins and O'Neal study (Robins, 1966), for example, found that "the clinic psychiatric diagnosis was disappointing" but "the social history, medical examination, and psychological tests were so systematically collected that they lent themselves readily to research purposes" (p. 17). Even the sophisticated evaluation procedures of the child guidance clinics of the Jewish Board of Guardians provided only "information from the social case records, including psychiatric and psychological reports" for their childhood ratings (Lehrman et al., 1949). Without complete evaluation data available from childhood records, systematic comparison of childhood and adult behavior is severely limited.

3. *Inconsistency in the data which was included in the evaluation.*

Mednick and McNeil (1968) point out the inherent disadvantage of trying to trace the illness of the adult back to childhood where the researcher has to content himself with whatever childhood data he can obtain, data likely to be "insufficient at its source" and inconsistent across child subjects. This latter inconsistency may lead to gross errors in specifying the childhood characteristics which are related to a particular outcome in adulthood. For example, if all the adults under study have not been checked, as children, on the *same* list of behaviors, or were not administered the *same* battery of tests, the childhood behavior or personality characteristic that seems, from the study, to be related to a certain adult outcome may simply not have been *considered* in the childhood assessment of others in the sample.

4. *Lack of equivalence between data collected at the two assessment points: Referral and Follow-up.*

Previous studies have compared various kinds of childhood data with various other kinds of follow-up data, such as parent's report of childhood behavior compared with psychiatric interview of this child grown up (Schofield and Balian, 1959; Stabenau and Pollen, 1970). The lack of equivalence in the two sets of comparison data is, of course, largely a result of the "post hoc" planning in the studies and, to a lesser degree, of the actual change in the applicability of some assessment items from childhood, for example, that of "school behavior;" to the adult evaluation. If the prospect for a follow-up is built into the childhood assessment techniques, the latter can be standardized so that data can be compared with adult reevaluation.

5. *Lack of attempt to predict adult outcome for each individual child.*

Some previous studies have formulated hypotheses as to the *group* characteristics they might expect in their follow-up sample, for example, the greater probability of sociopathic adulthood in a group of children referred for behavior problems (Glueck and Glueck, 1959; Robins, 1966; Morris et al., 1956), the greater likelihood of psychoses and other psychiatric illness in children of psychotic parents (Anthony, 1968; Mednick and Schulsinger, 1970), the expectation of delinquency in children of broken homes (Lehrman et al., 1949).

What still needs to be done, however, is to predict social adjustment and the kind of severity of adult disturbance *for a particular child* from the data of his early evaluation. This kind of individualized and discriminative prediction is difficult to do and would seem to require, at least, a comprehensive, in-depth study of many facets of the child, including behavior, psychological assets and liabilities, conflicts and means of defense, and the strengths and weaknesses within his social environment.

OBJECTIVES

The first of three main objectives of this study was to determine whether overall social and personal adjustment of some 200 adults who were seen as children at the Washington University Child Guidance Clinic in 1961-65 can be predicted from behavior symptoms and social data collected consistently on each child and from ratings made from the child's clinical evaluation data.

A second main objective was to determine which of the behavioral, social, and personality variables of childhood are associated with degree and kind of disturbance in adulthood, that is, to develop patterns of childhood variables which are significant for adult adjustment.

A third objective was to evaluate the influence of therapy on adult outcome of adjustment and on the accuracy of the predictions made from childhood data. For this purpose, follow-up data of the groups of treated and untreated children were compared.

DESIGN OF THE RESEARCH

This research was designed to test the assumption that social and personal adjustment in young adulthood can be predicted from behaviors, symptoms, social adjustment, personality variables, and family characteristics of childhood. It consists of a follow-up of a sample of 200 children who had been referred to a child guidance clinic with a wide variety of emotional and behavior disorders, that is, a comprehensive "high risk" sample; the data are consistent across all child subjects and were obtained in a form subject to quantification and coding; the predictions from childhood are made for each child on the basis of his individual and family characteristics and related to his social and personal adjustment in adulthood.

The high risk design provides its own control group as several recent writers have pointed out (Mednick and McNeil, 1968). In the present design, the experimental group comprises those subjects who are found to be poorly adjusted in adulthood, and the controls are the subjects who were also referred to child guidance as children but who did *not* show adult maladjustment. The effort was then made to specify the childhood variables that differentiate these two groups. The variable of therapeutic intervention could also be taken into account since some of each group, those who became maladjusted adults and those who did not, had received therapy in childhood.

A number of factors make the Washington University Child Guidance Clinic particularly well suited for an in-depth follow-up study. This clinic has had a continuous and stable existence since 1947. It serves the needs of a large metropolitan area and children from all social classes are referred for a variety of disorders, from simple bothersome habits through learning disorders, anxiety states, phobias, antisocial behavior, and psychosis. During the entire period of its existence, the clinic has operated in a tri-disciplinary approach to diagnosis and treatment of the child-within-his-family. For over 25 years, standard diagnostic materials, including social history, school reports, psychiatric interviews, and a consistent battery of psychological tests, have been collected on some 100 to 200 children each year. A diagnostic conference was held about each child and a diagnostic formulation recorded. About half the children received treatment.

In 1960 when plans were initiated for this prospective follow-up study, a system of data collection was set up to insure consistency across all children in assessment. From then on, an application form, symptom and behavior checklist, and developmental questionnaire were administered for each child.

Another advantage in drawing upon the children seen at the Washington University Child Guidance Clinic is the accessibility of subjects for follow-up. This study, like the Robins and O'Neal study (Robins, 1966), followed a St. Louis group of children. Even though the subjects were followed up 30 years after they were seen in the St. Louis City Child Guidance Clinic, Robins and O'Neal located 88% of these former patients and about half of the original total were still in St. Louis. In the present study, of 342 adults who had been referred as children in 1961-65 and who met the criteria for inclusion in the sample (described later), 286, or 84% were located.

PROCEDURES

The subjects were assessed in person at two points in time: the first was during the childhood diagnostic evaluation which was part of the service offered to those referred to the Child Guidance Clinic; the second consisted of interviews with the subjects and, separately, with their mothers some 10 to 15 years after their child guidance contact. The project was planned to take advantage of the full clinical evaluation which is regularly done at the Clinic. The findings from these evaluations are the basis for dynamic formulation of the personality and for an understanding of problems the child is presenting, for the diagnosis and estimate of seriousness of disturbance, and for the recommendations including decisions about therapy which are presented to the parents.

As Kohlberg points out (Kohlberg et al., p. 1272), few attempts have been made to test, through follow-up research, the usefulness of psychodynamic *clinical* findings to predict to adult outcome. This effort was made in this research although the difficulty in subjecting clinical process to objectivity was duly recognized. In addition to the records of the clinical process, also collected at the time of child guidance referral were the applications, symptom and developmental "forms" filled out by parents, and the school reports from teachers.

The procedures at follow-up in young adulthood provided much less data. Judgments as to social and personal adjustment were based on one interview with the subject and one with his or her mother. "Factual" data were recorded also from these two interviews. This limitation was imposed by the lack of sufficient funding. As originally planned, clinical evaluation of the subjects would have been repeated on a select sample to evaluate *intrapsychic* status as well as the more overt indices of adjustment and, thus, to provide consistency between data at childhood and adulthood.

Procedures Applied to Childhood Data

The measures used at the time of Clinic contact were designed to provide a full picture of the child, both behaviorally and intrapsychically, and of the child within family and school settings. They included the following forms administered during the intake process and the clinical assessment techniques of the diagnostic evaluation (Appendix A).

Forms

1. *Application Form.* This form was filled out by the parents (usually mother) and contains a wealth of information, some 72 items in all, consisting of demographic data, details about the referral and problems as perceived, family characteristics, such as composition, mobility, and employment data.

2. *Symptom List.* This form was developed to provide information which would be consistent across all children as to the specific symptoms and behavior the child was displaying at the time of referral. Filled out by the parents, it contains 38 items, each arranged in 4 degrees of severity with numerous examples of behavior at each level of severity. Parents were asked to underline specific behaviors that applied to their child.

3. *Developmental Questionnaire.* This 86-item questionnaire filled out by the parents consists mainly of checklists in terms of events and parental attitudes considered important in early development.

4. *School Report.* This form was given to the parents at time of intake to pass on to their school principal who then had the child's teacher fill it out and send it back directly to the Clinic. It contains factual information as to the results of tests, IQ, and achievement, which were administered at school; special educational placement and subjective data such as the teacher's estimate of the child's working up to capacity, a 31-item checklist as to the problems she perceives at school and a discursive description of the child's functioning at school.

Much of the form data were already in quantitative form and had only to be coded by the project researchers. Coding categories were developed for the discursive responses.

Diagnostic Evaluation at Clinic

Parents were seen together for an Intake interview at the Clinic and at this time a decision was made as to whether or not they would be offered a diagnostic appraisal. If it was offered and accepted, the diagnostic evaluation was conducted, on the average, a few weeks later. The parents were seen together and then separately for social history; a psychologist administered a standard battery of tests to the child including at least a Wechsler or Stanford-Binet individual intelligence test, Rorschach, TAT, Bender or Beery Visuo-Motor test; a psychiatrist interviewed the child in two or three one-hour sessions.

This diagnostic process took place over the period of a week. Then, a diagnostic conference was held with each professional presenting his findings and discussing the dynamics, assets, and disabilities within the child and the family interrelationships, strengths, and weaknesses. Together the conference participants worked out a diagnostic formulation (based on Diagnostic Guidelines [Appendix A], and recommendations which the conference chairman recorded on a form. Including a postdiagnostic session held with the parents, the evaluation usually involved 8 or 9 contacts in all. If the child was taken into treatment, a record of this treatment was kept. (This latter material was not as consistently recorded as the form data.)

Rating of Clinical Data. The results of this diagnostic evaluation were in the child's record in the form of 1) an Intake Interview and a detailed social history, 2) a psychological test report and the actual protocols of each test, intelligence and projective, 3) process recording of psychiatric interviews, 4) the conference form filled in at the conference after the clinical evaluation and

5) process notes of treatment interviews. In order to achieve as much consistency in rating as possible, a set of researchers was employed at the time of the follow-up study to rate this material from childhood.

Psychological and Psychiatric Ratings (Appendix B). At follow-up a child psychiatrist, using the typescripts of the Clinic psychiatric interviews, rated each child on 12 personality variables, assigned a diagnostic label, and assessed the degree of severity of the disturbance. The same variables were rated independently by a clinical psychologist from test protocols.

Variables were based on psychoanalytic theory and were those usually addressed in psychological and psychiatric reports in the Clinic diagnostic process. Some are personality traits, such as aggressivity, emotionality, concreteness; others have to do with efficiency of psychological functioning, such as reality testing, logicality of thinking, coping; while still others reflect concepts central to psychoanalytic theory of dynamics, such as conflicts, degree of anxiety, and the nature and efficiency of defenses.

Most of these variables were rated on a 5-point scale of pathology comparable to that used in Social Adjustment ratings. Conflicts, defenses, and diagnosis were simply named but efficiency of defenses and overall severity of disturbance were rated on the 5-point scale. The psychologist and psychiatrist each had a manual for rating these personality variables with each of five steps on a continuum of severity defined for each variable (Appendix B).

This manual had been developed by psychologists of the Clinic[1] for use in E. James Anthony's research, "The Study of Children of Psychotic Parents" (MH 12043). Pilot studies in that project had led the psychologists to the conclusion that rating important *personality* variables on the basis of *all* the test data discriminated the experimental and control groups better than did discrete test data (scores, IQs, etc.). Psychiatrists in the research project used the same personality variables and defined them to suit psychiatric interview data.

Ratings of Social and Personal Adjustment (Appendix B). An experienced social worker, using social history and intake reports, made ratings on the child's social adjustment in five life areas of functioning, that is, within family, school performance, relationship to teachers, to peers, and in larger society. She also rated personal adjustment in areas of anxiety, defenses, self-concept, affect, object relationships, and moral development. This latter assessment was difficult to do and its validity is highly questionable since it was based only on reports of the parents and not on process from the child. Finally, she gave

---

[1] In addition to Loretta Cass, the other psychologists involved in developing the scales and variables were Marylyn Voerg, Larry Bass, Lois Franklin, and John B. Lewis.

each child an overall rating of life-adjustment of functioning. Social Adjustment and Personal Adjustment ratings were also made from the follow-up interviews and are described in detail in the next section.

Rating of Parent-Child Variables (Appendix B). In addition to rating social and personal adjustment of the child from intake and social history recordings, the research social worker also rated several parental and parent-child variables which were considered to be important to the child's adjustment. These were judgmental ratings done after reading intake and social history recordings and included the feelings of both parents about this child, the quality of discipline, their reaction to the child's problem, each parent's emotional stabiity and capacity to cope, and their relationship to one another. She also listed and rated the severity of trauma and constitutional factors which might have affected development.

The three research professionals, psychologist, psychiatrist, and social worker, made their ratings independently from one another and without knowledge of the follow-up interviews.

Procedures at Follow-up

A project coordinator, employed specifically for this research, went through child guidance records from June 1, 1961, to October 31, 1965, in sequence, selecting those children who met the criteria for follow-up. They were to be 17 years of age or older at follow-up, have IQ of 75 or higher, have undergone a full diagnostic evaluation, and have completed forms and diagnostic data in the file. Of the children referred to the clinic during the period designated, 342 met these criteria.

Contacting and Interviewing Subjects. The project coordinator located 286, or 84%, of the 342 potential subjects, a figure near to that of the Robins study. The coordinator first tried to call the parents using the address listed in the childhood record, and, if a parent answered, she explained the project and sought the cooperation of the parents and the phone number and address of their child if he or she was no longer at home. Many families who had moved were still listed in the telephone book or city directory.

If the parents could not be found in this way, various other techniques were employed. Using the address in the record, the coordinator consulted the city and county directory in the year of child guidance referral to locate those neighbors of the family in that year who were listed also in current directories. These neighbors were contacted and several out-of-town families were found through their cooperation. Other sources of information were labor unions, professional organizations, and service records. Most interviews were arranged by telephone; a letter was sent when the subjects could not be reached by phone and to confirm appointments once cooperation had been promised

Of the 286 families who could be located, 257 were actually contacted. The other 29 were not, primarily because of the distance involved or the difficulty in reaching them by phone. Of those contacted, 202, or 78.6%, agreed to participate. Refusal to participate came from parents of 18 potential subjects and from 31 of the grown-up children. Another 5 potential subjects agreed to participate but failed to keep scheduled appointments. One subject had died. Reasons for refusals were varied and included parents' feelings about the Clinic, their wish that their children not be bothered, and the subjects' lack of interest or lack of time. In 10 of the instances of refusal there was strong opposition to participation. A reasonable attempt was always made to gain cooperation but the effort was terminated when it seemed to be futile.

Of the 202 subjects who agreed to participate, 200 were interviewed. Of these, 111 (55.5%) lived in suburban St. Louis, 37 (18.5%) in St Louis city, 20 (10%) in outlying areas of Missouri, and 32 (16%) in other states.[2] Mothers of 190 of the subjects were also interviewed, separately from their offspring, and data were obtained independently from each interviewee. Of the 10 mothers not interviewed, 8 refused to participate, and 2 were not seen because of geographic location.

Once an appointment had been made for the interviews, one or two of the research staff went to the home of the subject and of his mother to conduct the interviews. A few persons (about 2%) were interviewed at the research center. Ten interviewers participated in the project: 6 psychologists, 2 child psychiatrists, 1 social worker, and the project coordinator. Most of the interviews, some 77%, were done by three of these interviewers, two psychologists and the coordinator. Two staff people interviewed together in the initial stages of the project, recorded their data separately, made independent ratings, and established reliability for the ratings (Appendix C). Each interviewer who came on to the project went through this learning process. The subject and mother were interviewed separately so that no collusion was possible. Sometimes they were in different cities.

Follow-up Measures

Data Recorded from Interview. Two kinds of data were recorded at the time of the interviews and both kinds were obtained from the subject and, independently, from the mother.

1. *Guideline data* (Appendix C).

The interviewer, using a form devised for the purpose, recorded factual information such as the subject's age, marital status, children, living arrangements and moves, educational and occupational data, health and hospitaliza-

[2]The Grant Foundation provided travel and supplementary salary funds.

tion, court contacts, drug and liquor usage, and service record. In addition to these same items pertaining to the subject, mother was asked for information about her other children, especially in regard to any special educational or psychiatric help that they had needed. This "guideline" information was categorized for coding.

  2. *Essay part of interview* (Appendix C).

In addition to this factual information, the subject and mother were each asked about 1) the subject's functioning in predetermined areas such as in school or at work, in relationship with siblings, parents, friends and spouse, in heterosexual relationships; 2) whether or not he had sought other mental health services since his childhood referral to the Clinic and if he had, the details of this service; 3) his recollection of the clinic service in detail; 4) his present self-concept; 5) crises that might have occurred since his clinic referral and 6) what he would change about his life if he were able to do so. In the mother's case, these questions were in reference to the *subject's* behavior and attitudes except for the item asking for recollections about the clinic service where her opinions were also recorded. This "essay" part of the interview was recorded in detail for each area and later typed.

Assessments Based on Interview Data. As soon as possible after the interview, each interviewer filled out three forms containing judgments about the subject

  1. *Impressions of the subject's psychological functioning.*

The interviewer recorded his (clinical) impressions on prescribed items of functioning such as the subject's nervousness, openness, tendency to deny or project, carefulness, emotionality and impulsivity, trust of the interviewer and of those in his environment, and respect for the rights of others.

  2. *Rating of social adjustment.*

Using all the information gained from interviewing the subject and mother, the interviewer rated the subject's life functioning in five areas (Items A through E): within family, school, and/or job, relationship with teachers or boss, relationship to peers, and relationships in larger society. In each of these areas, the rating was on a scale from 1 to 5 (1= good adjustment and the absence of problems; 3= moderately serious problems; 5= incapacitating degree of problem behavior). Behavioral examples are provided for each point on the rating scale.

  Then a rating was made of overall life adjustment LAR (Item F) which was a kind of global assessment (1 =good overall functioning; 5=incapacitating maladjustment). For ratings 2 through 5, possible diagnostic labels are suggested but the interviewer was not expected to do an actual clinical diagnosis in those cases where he thought he did not have enough information to do so. This "global" rating and the sum of social adjustment (ASSA) ratings (sum of Items A through E) were both used as criteria of adult outcome. They could be compared with ratings on the same scale made from childhood data by the social worker (CSSA).

3. Rating of personal adjustment.

Using the interview material, both factual and impressionistic, the interviewer also rated the subject in Personal Adjustment. This form consisted of six psychological variables: anxiety, defenses, self-concept, appropriateness and degree of affect, capacity for object relationships, and moral and ethical development. Each variable was rated on a scale from 1 to 5 (1 = health; 5=incapacitation in that area). Descriptions of the behavioral referents were provided for each point on the scale.

Repeat Administration of Symptom List. The interviewer asked the subject and mother each to fill out and send back to the project coordinator a symptom list which was the same as that which the mother had filled out at the time of clinic contact except for a few changes in wording to suit adult status (e.g., resistance to work instead of to school). Of the 200 pairs interviewed, 85 subjects and 71 mothers returned these forms. Of these, in 51 cases both the mother and her grown-up child returned the forms and in 69 cases mothers had filled in the symptom list for their children both at time of clinic contact and at follow-up.

RESULTS

The sample for this study was drawn from the files of the Washington University Child Guidance Clinic. Some characteristics of the sample were influenced by the Clinic's policies and its role in the community since these factors had some effect on the type of children who were referred. This clinic provided services to parents and children from infancy to 18 years of age who lived in St. Louis city, its suburbs, and surrounding small towns. There were no income restrictions and fees were charged on a sliding scale.

In addition to providing direct services, the Clinic is a major training center for mental health professionals of various disciplines. Although located in the inner city, this university clinic attracted a varied client group including those who were psychiatrically sophisticated. At the time the subjects came to the Clinic relatively few inner city residents were aware that the Clinic could be a resource for them.

The types of children referred to the Clinic were also influenced by the availability of similar services. Three other child guidance clinics existed in the region at the time, one serving primarily court referred children and youth, one serving mainly Catholic families, and one serving suburban families with low to moderate incomes. The children seen at the Washington University Clinic included relatively few acting out or delinquent youngsters in contrast to the well-known Robins follow-up study done at a municipal clinic in St. Louis. None of the subjects of the present study were court referred, while 22% were referred by parents, 41% by physicians or mental health professionals, and 19% by schools.

The proportion of Catholic children in the sample, 26%, was somewhat lower than that of the Catholic population in the St. Louis area and this discrepancy was partially accounted for by the existence of a clinic serving mainly Catholic families. Of the subjects, 52% were Protestant, 12% Jewish, and 6% of other religions.

The sample selected according to the criteria outlined earlier in "Procedures at Follow-Up" was fairly representative of the Clinic population, except for the exclusion of children with IQs under 75. Several specific characteristics of the sample selected and of those children remaining in the potential subject pool were compared. There were no significant differences in the two groups in relation to sex, reason they came to the clinic, diagnosis, or severity of disturbance. The mean IQ of the sample was slightly higher than those not participating and there was a significant difference in age ($X^2 = 7.85$, $p < .05$) with the sample containing more children 5 years old or younger and fewer children 12 years and older, than those who met the sample criteria but did not participate in the study.

Description of Subjects in Childhood

Demographic Characteristics

The 200 subjects, as they were in childhood, are described in terms of demographic data, parental characteristics, and developmental history, and from the perspective of parents, teachers, and clinicians.

The modal child in this study was a white, Protestant, 9-year-old male from a lower middle class, home owning, intact family with 3 children. Of the subjects, 74% were male and 26% female. The mean age was 9.4 years. Their ages, by sex, at the time of Clinic application are presented in Table 1.

As can be seen in Table 1, most (71%) of the children included in the sample came to the Clinic during the latency period of development (6 through 11 years). The oldest subject at time of evaluation was 15 years, and 22.5% of the subjects were 12 to 15 years old. There was no significant difference in the age of boys and girls at the time they first came to the Clinic. The first born child in a family was more likely to come to the Clinic than those in other ordinal positions: 46% of the subjects were first born, 31% second born, 13% third born, and the remaining 10% were born fourth to ninth in their families.

Table 1. Sex and Age of Children at Time of Clinic Application

Age (in years)[a]	Male		Female		Both Sexes	
	N	%	N	%	N	%
1-5	9	6.0	3	5.9	12	6.0
6-8	53	35.6	18	35.2	71	35.5
9-11	56	37.6	16	31.4	72	36.0
12-15	31	20.8	14	27.5	45	22.5
Total	149	100.0	51	100.0	200	100.0

[a] $X^2=1.8$, no significant differences in ages of girls and boys.

The sample contained only 15 (7.5%) black children, slightly fewer than expected on the basis of the potential subject pool. Ten percent (34) of the potential subjects were black and the remaining 90% white. It was more difficult to locate blacks than whites, partly because of the rapid movement of people away from the inner city and the destruction of living accommodations in the city.[3] Although many more white subjects than black subjects participated in the study, the two groups did not differ significantly in the proportion who agreed to participate once located.

At Clinic referral, all but 4.7% of the subjects were in school. Forty-three percent were in the first 3 grades, 32.8% in grades 4 through 6, and 18.5% in junior or senior high school. One subject was in a special class, but all the others were in regular classrooms in public or parochial schools.

Family Characteristics

Certain family characteristics are presented to provide information about the family environment of the subjects in childhood. These children came from relatively stable, intact, functioning families in which fathers worked and mothers were not employed. Of the children, 75% were being reared by both natural parents, 7% by a parent and stepparent, and 11% by mothers alone. Of the remainder, six children lived with a parent and a relative, one with foster parents and eight were adopted. Data at follow-up regarding parents' marital status were not systematically obtained, but some separations and divorces had occurred since the initial Clinic contact. Thus, some children experienced family instability following initial contact with the Clinic, which suggests that families did not remain as stable as they appeared at time of application.

[3] The Clinic population has changed dramatically since the early 1960s and now nearly 50% of the Clinic patients are black.

Seventy percent of the families owned their own one or two family homes, 14% rented houses, and 11% rented apartments. This high rate of home ownership suggested family stability and adequate income levels. Families had lived an average of 3.6 places between the time of the child's birth and Clinic contact, although 44% were living in their present residence, or had made only one move, since the child's birth. Families varied in size with a range of 1 to 9 children (mean: 3.2). Grandparents had lived in the homes of 40% of the subjects during some part of their lives.

Fathers tended to be older than mothers with a mean age of 39 years and an age range of 27 to 71 years. The mean age of mothers was 36 years and the range was 23 to 59 years.

Most (96%) fathers were employed full time. Only three fathers were un-employed, four worked part time, and the rest worked 40 or more hours per week with 24% working over 51 hours per week. Sixty-two percent of the fathers were in white collar or professional positions, 21% were skilled labor-ers, and 15% were in semi- or unskilled jobs.

The educational level of these fathers corresponded to their occupational status. Their education ranged from completion of third grade to completion of doctoral degrees; 69% had at least a high school degree. Bachelors, masters or doctoral degrees were obtained by 21% of the fathers.

In contrast to the fathers, most mothers were not employed; 71% were full time housewives, 14% worked part time, and 14% worked full time. There was little difference in the educational levels of mothers and fathers. Mothers' education ranged from completion of fifth grade to completion of the doctoral degree; 65% had at least a high school degree. The socioeconomic status of these families, based on the Hollingshead-Redlick Index was as follows: Level I: 13%; Level II: 16%; Level III: 49%; Level IV: 15%; Level V: 7%.

Parents' emotional stability and coping capacities were rated on a 5-point scale from their social histories recorded during Clinic service. Six percent of the mothers and 15.5% of the fathers were rated as fairly mature and well ad-justed while the rest were rated as moderately or severely disturbed or unsta-ble. Even fewer parents were rated as having adequate coping capacity: 1.5% of the mothers and 2.5% of the fathers. Marital relationship ratings were also quite negative. Five percent of the couples were rated as having good relation-ships, while 41% received ratings of moderate conflict and 31% serious con-flict; the remaining 22% were rated as wholly incompatible, and in most instances were divorced or separated. In seven families one parent was dead.

Children's Developmental History

Information about pregnancy, birth, neonatal condition, and infant devel-opment was obtained from parents at the time of Clinic contact. Pregnancies were normal with no complications for 40% of the subjects. Twenty-nine per-cent had one complication and 31% two or more complications. The most fre-quent complications were nausea (26%), swelling (14%), accidents (10)%, and bleeding (10%), while other complications such as anemia and Rh factor were reported for less than 10% of the subjects.

A wide variety of emotionally stressful events during pregnancy were reported by 42% of the mothers; the most frequent was marital conflict (8%). Seventy-two percent of the mothers stated they were happy about their pregnancy and accepted it.

For 98% of the subjects there were one or more complications at birth; the most frequent was prolonged labor, 11 or more hours (30%). Eleven percent of the deliveries were induced and 21% were by instrument. Eleven percent of the subjects were in incubators while 9% weighed less than 5 pounds at birth.

Some subjects experienced mild difficulties in the first year of life: 23% had difficulty with formula; 20%, moderate or severe colic; 11%, elimination difficulties; 16%, some difficulty with nursing. Along with these difficulties, 60% of the parents reported stressful family events during the child's first year. The most frequent stresses were marital conflict (13%), illness in the family (13%), and financial problems (7%).

In infancy and early childhood a few children showed some unusual behavior such as rocking (15%), bed shaking (8%), and head banging (7%).

Some traumatic events such as operations, accidents, and parental absenses were experienced by 79% of the subjects. Seventy-nine percent had one or more operations (this, however, includes circumcision), 53% had one or more accidents, 19% experienced the prolonged absence of a parent, usually the father, prior to age 6, and 4% lost a parent through death. All but 13% of the subjects had one or more serious illnesses during early childhood, but the nature and severity of the illnesses were not known.

Parents' Perception of Children's Problems

Parents' perceptions of their children's difficulties were obtained from forms filled out by the parents (Appendix A). It was evident that parents noticed their children having problems at an earlier age than the age at which they brought them to the Clinic. For example, parents, or other people in contact with these children, recognized problems in 74 children before age 6, but only 12 children were brought to the Clinic prior to age 6. Most parents (72%) did not initiate Clinic contact until it was suggested by someone else. The major sources of referral to the Clinic were social agencies and mental health professionals (22%), physicians (19%), and schools (19%). There were some significant differences between boys and girls in relation to referral sources ($X^2 = 13.07$, $p < .02$). A higher proportion of girls (42%) than boys (22.7%) came to the Clinic at the suggestion of parents. In contrast, schools referred only 5.8% of the girls, but 23.4% of the boys came at the suggestion of schools. There were no significant relationships between referral sources and age at referral.

The major reasons parents gave for bringing their children to the Clinic were behavior problems (36%) and poor school achievement (27.5%) (Table 2). Thus, parental or referral source concerns about poor achievement

Table 2.   Primary Reasons for Referral to Clinic According to Parents

Reasons	N	%
Poor school achievement	55	27.5
Behavior problem at home	40	20.0
Behavior problem outside home	32	16.0
Fearful-anxious	20	10.0
Withdrawal and somatic complaints	16	8.0
Trouble with peers	9	4.5
Hyperactive	5	2.5
Other	21	10.5
No information	2	1.0

and bad behavior were more likely to bring children to the Clinic than anxious, withdrawn, or fearful behavior (18%). Only 5 children, all boys, came to the Clinic because of hyperactivity. There were no significant age or sex differences in relation to reasons children were brought to the Clinic.

Symptoms. In contrast to the few behavioral difficulties reported for the first year of life, parents indicated a considerable number of behavior difficulties as the child grew older. Parents completed a 38-item symptom list at time of application (Appendix A). Each item on the list describes child behaviors and parents underlined the specific behaviors characteristic of their child. On the symptom list, children had a mean of 18 symptoms checked, while the number of symptoms ranged from 0 to 32. The behaviors listed for each symptom were grouped into four degrees of seriousness (minimal, mild, moderate, and severe), and could be weighted 1, 2, 3, or 4 according to the behaviors underlined by the parents.

When the symptoms were weighted and the sum of each child's *weighted* symptoms computed, the mean for the children's sample was 35.66±15.22 out of a possible weighted symptom sum of 152 (4 degrees of seriousness for each of 38 symptoms). Few children showed the most severe behavior described and 75% of the children showed minimal or no disturbance on almost half (18) of the symptoms. The number of children reported to show the most severely disturbed behavior varied from 0 to 20 on different items. However, except for all but hyperactivity (16), resistance (20), and rebelliousness with adults (16), the frequencies in the most disturbed categories were 6 or less.

The frequencies with which parents reported that specific symptoms were present varied from 5 to 88% as shown in Table 3.

Although more children experienced eating difficulties than any other symptom, 46% of them showed only mild difficulty as described on the symptom list: "Has a few food dislikes, but generally eats well; occasionally skips meals or overeats." From the behavioral description it is evident that this type

Table 3. Parents' Report of Children's Symptoms

Symptom	Frequency N	Frequency %[a]	Age F ratio	Age p	Sex F ratio	Sex p
Eating difficulties	173	88			8.31	.004
Resistance	156	81				
Impulsive	156	80				
Hyperactive	154	78				
Aggressive	149	77	2.96	.033		
Sleep difficulties	148	76	3.43	.018		
Lying	145	74				
Depression	142	73				
Poor self-esteem	140	72				
Learning difficulties	139	71			7.06	.008
Restless	139	71			4.34	.037
Poor peer relations	130	66				
Rebellious	128	65				
Fantasy	125	64	3.93	.010		
Dependence	122	62				
Suspicious	111	57				
Antisocial acting out	99	51				
Fears	96	49				
Compulsive	94	48	3.26	.022	5.99	.015
School absence	92	46				
Bizarre behavior	91	46				
Stomach pain	87	44				
Reaction to change	84	43			5.39	.020
Poor coordination	68	35				
Stealing	66	34				
Thumb sucking	65	33				
Fears	64	33				
Respiratory	52	27				
Somatic	54	27				
Stutters	52	26				
Enuresis	51	26				
Retarded	48	24				
Masturbation	45	23				
Accident prone	42	22				
Heart symptoms	31	16				
Soiling	32	16	3.86	.010		
Visual-hearing	26	13				
Urinary	10	5				

[a]Size of sample on which percentage is based varies because of missing data.
[b]ANOVA, F ratio and p values given.

of eating behavior is fairly normal, so the finding of high incidence of eating difficulties can be discounted. The next most frequently reported behaviors— resistance, impulsivity, hyperactivity, and aggressivity—are the kinds of things particularly annoying to other people and consequently likely to be noticed by parents. The least frequently reported symptoms were related to physical problems and functions such as urinary problems and enuresis, respiratory and heart difficulties; speech, visual, and hearing difficulties.

There were significant age differences in the severity of five symptoms: the youngest children (4-5 years) showed more disturbance in sleeping, fantasy, and aggressive behavior; whereas soiling was most severe in the 6-8-year-old group; and compulsive behavior was most severe in the youngest (4-5) and oldest (12-15) age groups. Sex differences were noted in five symptoms. Females showed more severe disturbance ratings than males in eating, reaction to change, and compulsive behavior. Males had more serious disturbance ratings in the areas of learning problems and restless behavior.

There were some differences between parents' reports of their children's symptomatic behavior and their account of the primary reason for bringing the child to the Clinic. For example, only 3% of the children were brought to the Clinic primarily because of hyperactivity, but 78% were described on the symptom list as hyperactive. Similarly, 28% came to the Clinic mainly because of school difficulties, but 72% of the children were experiencing some difficulties in school according to the detailed symptom checklist.

In summary, the subjects showed little disturbed behavior in infancy but by the time they came to the Clinic their parents indicated many symptoms of disturbance including symptoms of an acting out, aggressive, impulsive, rebellious nature as well as those of withdrawal, depression, fears, and anxiety.

Parents' Attitudes Toward Their Child

Parents' attitudes toward their child at time of Clinic contact were rated on a 5-point scale. Of the mothers, 72% were rated as quite dissatisfied with the child, 13% somewhat dissatisfied, 12% actively rejecting, and only 3% accepting. Fathers were rated as significantly more accepting than mothers; 8% were accepting, 55% somewhat dissatisfied, 32% quite dissatisfied, and 5% actively rejecting ($X^2 = 86.94$, $p < .001$).

Parents' reaction to the child's problems were also rated. Only 4% of the parents were rated as being able to see their part in the child's problems while 58% viewed the problem as something bad within the child, and 39% viewed the problem as the child's unwillingness to conform.

In view of these negative findings it was interesting to note that, at follow-up, a few mothers commented that they had not thought there was much wrong with the child when he was taken to the Clinic, but rather that they didn't know how to cope or were having problems themselves.

Teachers' Perceptions of the Children

At the time of Clinic contact, teachers were sent a form on which they were asked to indicate the presence or absense of 31 behavior items for each child. All items but two were problem behaviors. The exceptions were leadership qualities (11 children) and exceptional brightness (14 children). As can be seen in Table 4, the most frequently reported problem behaviors were those that clearly interfered with the child's school functioning: difficulty concentrating (60%), restlessness (50%), daydreaming (42%), and inability to get along with other children (32%). In addition to behavior suggesting difficulty in attending to the task of learning, about one fourth of the children showed acting out behavior: disobedience (28%), temper (24%), resistance to authority (22%), and fighting (20%). Other types of difficult behavior such as nail biting, selfishness, and speech difficulties were infrequent. A few children were depressed (17%) and withdrawn (21%).

The average number of behavior difficulties reported by teachers was 4.8 from the checklist of 31, somewhat less, proportionately, than the average of 18 from the checklist of 38 reported by parents. Thirteen behavior items on the teachers' checklist were similar to the parents' symptom list. On all 13 items parents more frequently than teachers reported that the children showed such behavior. For example, 32% of the children had difficulty with other children according to teachers, and 66% according to parents; teachers reported that 22% of the children were resistant, while 81% were so identified by parents.

There were no significant differences in the *total* number of behaviors reported for boys and girls nor for different age groups. However, there were sex differences in the frequency with which specific symptoms were checked. Three symptoms were more frequently checked for girls than boys. These were "withdraws from other children" ($X^2 = 9.89$, 1 df, $p < .002$), "physical complaints" ($X^2 = 5.61$, 1 df, $p < .02$), and "unusual fears" ($X^2 = 4.93$, 1 df, $p < .05$).

Age effects were evident for five items. Younger children were more frequently rated as having difficulty concentrating ($t = 3.20$, 185 df, $p < .01$), resistant to authority ($t = 2.76$, 185 df, $p < .01$), and thumb sucking ($t = 2.49$, 185 df, $p < .02$). Children who were identified as depressed ($t = 2.87$, 185 df, $p .01$) and truant ($t = 3.32$, 185 df, $p < .01$) tended to be older.

Clinicians' View of Children

The information obtained during the Clinic evaluation provided the basis for assigning subjects to diagnostic categories, for rating subjects' childhood disturbance, and for rating their social adjustment (Appendix).

Children were assigned to one of 10 diagnostic categories derived from the GAP classification system. Each child received three diagnoses: one made currently by a psychiatrist on the basis of childhood psychiatric interviews,

Table 4. Teachers' Report of Children's Problems

Problems	Frequencies		Differences			
	N	%	Age [a]		Sex [b]	
			t	p	X²	p
Difficulty in concentrating	113	60	3.20	.01		
Restlessness	93	50				
Daydreaming	79	42				
Fails to get along with other children	59	32				
Disobedient	52	28				
Slow in learning to do things	49	26				
Temper display	45	24				
Resistant to authority	42	22	2.76	.01		
Withdraws from other children	40	21			9.89	.002
Fighting	38	20				
Depressed	32	17	2.87	.01		
Lying	30	16				
Boastful	28	15				
Speech defect	27	14				
Physical complaints	22	12			5.61	.02
Unusual fears	20	11			4.93	.05
Nail biting	18	10				
Selfish	17	9				
Exceptional brightness	14	7				
Prefers younger children	14	7				
Leadership qualities	11	6				
Stealing	10	5				
Bed or clothes wetting	8	4				
Sleep disturbances	8	4				
Truant from home or school	7	4	3.32	.01		
Prefers to play with opposite sex	7	4				
Feeding problem	6	3				
Sex misbehavior	5	3				
Lack of bowel control	5	3				
Thumb or finger sucking	5	3	2.49	.02		
Compulsive attacks	1	1				

[a] t test, 185 df.
[b] X², Yates correction, 1 df.

one made by a psychologist on the basis of psychological test protocols, and one which had been made in the Clinic by the diagnostic conference chairman at the end of a conference in which each professional presented and discussed his findings from the study of the child and his family.

Similarly, the severity of subjects' childhood disturbance was rated by three different judges—a psychiatrist, a psychologist, on the research team—and the diagnostic conference chairman. A 5-point scale was used (1 = healthy; 5 = incapacitating disturbance). Each child's social adjustment in childhood was also rated on a similar 5-point scale. The assessment of reliability of these ratings is described in Appendix C.

Clinical Diagnosis. There was not always agreement between the psychiatric, psychological, and diagnostic conference judgments as to a child's diagnosis. There was agreement in all three judgments for 58 subjects, agreement in two of three judgments for 98 additional subjects, and lack of agreement for 44 subjects (22%).

Two factors contributed to the lack of agreement in diagnostic judgments. Due to missing data only 2 diagnostic judgments were available for 24 of the subjects: diagnostic conference judgments were missing for 2 subjects and psychiatric judgments were missing for 22 subjects. Secondly, between the time of clinic evaluation (1961-1965) and the time of follow-up (1975-1977) there was a change in one category in the diagnostic classifications. The diagnostic conference classification system utilized a category of "neurotic behavior disorder" which was not utilized in the psychiatric and psychological diagnostic judgments made on the basis of the more recently developed GAP categories. Instead, the GAP classification included a category of "tension discharge disorder."

To examine the extent of agreement in diagnostic judgments, we reclassified the neurotic behavior disorders and the tension discharge disorders as personality disorders. There is some question about the reclassification of subjects originally in these two categories. The category "neurotic behavior disorder" seemed to include some children who might be classified as neurotic in the newer GAP system and others who might appropriately be classified as personality disorders.

We consider neurotic behavior disorder to be a meaningful category and, therefore, present the diagnostic conference judgments in Table 5 to describe the subjects' childhood diagnosis.

Half of the subjects were diagnosed neurotic, 15% personality disorder, 12% neurotic behavior disorder, 9.5% borderline psychosis or psychotic, and the remaining 13.5% in other categories as shown in Table 5. Boys and girls did not differ in diagnosis nor were there age differences in relation to diagnosis. There were significant differences in ratings of children's social adjustment (CSSA) for the different diagnostic categories with developmental and

Table 5.   Childhood Diagnosis from Diagnostic Conference

	Frequencies	
Diagnosis	N = 200	%
Normal	1	0.5
Developmental	10	5.0
Neurotic reaction	100	50.0
Neurotic behavior disorder	24	12.0
Personality disorder	30	15.0
Borderline psychosis	15	7.5
Psychosis	4	2.0
Mental deficiency	2	1.0
Brain syndrome	10	5.0
Psychophysical	2	1.0
Missing data	2	1.0

neurotic disorders below the mean and neurotic behavior disorders, personality disorders, and borderline psychosis all rated above the mean. The borderline group obtained the poorest social adjustment rating (see Table 11).

Emotional Disturbance. These subjects were judged to be quite disturbed in childhood, as is evident in the psychiatric, psychological, and diagnostic conference ratings of disturbance. Only one child was rated as healthy while at least 70% were rated as moderately or seriously disturbed by all three raters. As can be seen in Table 6, there were sharp differences among the raters in assessing the children's degree of disturbance (X^2 = 135.19, $p < .001$). The Clinic team tended to rate children at the extreme disturbance end of the scale, psychologists rated toward the middle, and psychiatrists tended more frequently to use the mild disturbance categories. Even though there were significant differences among the three different ratings, most of the children were rated at least moderately disturbed.

None of the three disturbance ratings showed differences between boys and girls. The only significant age difference was found in the *psychological ratings*. A higher percentage of the younger children, age 8 and under, than those 9-11 years or 12-15 years were rated in the two most severely disturbed categories (X^2 = 20.27, $p < .001$).

Social Adjustment. Subjects showed considerable difficulty in childhood social adjustment. As rated on a 5-point scale (Child Life Adjustment Rating/CLAR), 57% were moderately maladjusted, 36% were severely maladjusted, while 5% were mildly maladjusted and less than 2% were at the two ends of the scale—well adjusted and incapacitated.

Another measure of childhood social functioning was derived by summing the ratings on the five social adjustment items and thereby obtaining a score

Table 6. Children's Severity of Disturbance Ratings

Judge	Disturbance in Percent				
	Healthy	Mild	Moderate	Severe	Incapacitated
Diagnostic conf.	1	9	28	31	31
Psychological	1	10	53	35	1
Psychiatric	—	30	41	26	4

called the Childhood Sum of Social Adjustment (CSSA). The ratings on this variable ranged from 10 to 25 with a mean of 16.06 which is just on the more pathological side of moderate social maladjustment. There were no significant age or sex differences on either of these ratings.

In summary, ratings of subjects' childhood disturbance in two areas, personality disturbance and social adjustment, identified most of the subjects as moderately or severely disturbed in childhood and only one subject out of the 200 was rated as healthy. This finding was not surprising because all the children had been referred to or contacted the Clinic for help because of perceived behavioral and/or emotional problems.

Intelligence. The subjects' Full Scale Intelligence Quotient scores in childhood ranged from 75 to 141 and their distribution followed a normal curve. Fifteen percent of the subjects scored at the lower end of the distribution (75-89), 15% at the upper end of the distribution (120-141), 23% scored 90-99, 23% scored 100-109, and 24% scored 110-119. The mean scores were similar for Full Scale Intelligence Quotient (104.6), Verbal Quotient (104), and Performance Quotient (105). Thus, all but 15% of the subjects had average or above average IQ scores. The exclusion from the sample of children with IQs below 75 accounts for this mean above the 100 IQ average of the general population.

Correlation Between the Various Sources of Data as to Severity of Childhood Disturbance

Although there was a moderate amount of disagreement as to severity of disturbance in particular children among the three professions who rated the childhood data, their judgments and reports of symptoms and behaviors are, nevertheless, significantly correlated overall, as can be seen in Table 7.

In Table 7, some correlations pertain to two variables that were not truly independent. These are CSSA with CLAR and each of these with Personal Adjustment (PA). These ratings were made by the same person (social worker). The correlation between *number* of symptoms and the *weighted* total

Table 7. Intercorrelations Between the Major Disturbance Ratings in Childhood

Childhood Disturbance	Correlations[a]									
	CLAR	Sum PA	Po SCDR	Py SCDR	SCBR	INTENS	# Sympt	Wt. Sympt	FSIQ	SES
CSSA: Childhood sum of soc. adj. ratings	.639 ****	.462 ***	.172 **	.347 ****	.330 ****	.450 ****	.229 ****	.326 ****	-.247 ****	.213 ****
CLAR: Global life adj. ratings		.391 ****	.119 *	.215 ***	.222 ****	.402 ****	.193 **	.287 ****	-.159 *	.098
Sum PA: Sum of pers. adj. ratings			.135 *	.142 *	.150 *	.366 ****	.105	.156 *	-.083	.030
PoSCDR: Psychol. sum of disturb. ratings				.409 ****	.191 ***	.229 ****	.178 **	.199 ***	-.233 ****	.046
PySCDR: Psychiat. sum of disturb. ratings					.194 **	.297 ****	.163 *	.225 ***	-.264 ****	.127 *
SCBR: Total school behav. ratings						.171 *	.148	.147 *	-.169 *	.144 *
INTENS: Conf. ratings of disturb.							.106	.153 *	-.076	.150
#Symp.: Total number of symptoms								.906 ****	-.006	.016
Wt. Sympt.: Sum of weighted symptoms									-.065	.054 ****
FSIQ: Full scale intelligence quotient										.262

[a]Pearson r **** p < .001; *** p < .005; ** p < .01; * p < .05.

of these symptoms is expectedly high (.906). All the other correlations are between variables independently obtained. Of these the highest correlations were between social adjustment ratings and, respectively, the diagnostic conference rating of intensity of disturbance (r = .450), psychiatric disturbance rating (r = .347), total school behavior (r = .330), and weighted symptoms (r = .326). The independent psychiatric and psychological ratings were also highly correlated (r = .409). As can be seen from Table 7, the Clinic children were truly a "high risk" sample in that almost all of the assessments of their disturbance are significantly intercorrelated.

Follow-Up: The Children as Young Adults

The subjects at follow-up are described in terms of demographic characteristics, health, drug usage, and antisocial behavior. Their social and personal adjustment is presented in terms of ratings made by interviewers from information supplied by the subjects and their mothers. (Interview schedules and rating scales are reproduced in the Appendix.)

Demographic Characteristics

Subjects ranged from 17 to 28 years of age with a mean of 21 years. There were no significant differences in the age distribution of males and females. Of the subjects, 44% were 17 through 20 years old, 26% were 21 or 22 years old, and 29% were 23 through 28 years old. The sex distribution was 74% male and 26% female.

Most (72%) subjects were single, while 24% (47 subjects) were married and another 4% (8 subjects) were separated or divorced. The average age at marriage was 20 years. Marital status was not related to sex but was significantly related to age with 2% of those 17 to 20 married, 30% of those 21 and 22 years of age married, and 57% of those 23 to 28 years of age married ($X^2 = 58.52$, 2 df, p < .001). Thirty-two subjects had children; 21 had one child and 11 had 2 children. The children's ages ranged from 1 to 10 with an average of 3.2 years. Female subjects were more likely to be parents than male subjects ($X^2 = 7.384$, 1 df, p < .006).

Employment, Education, and Occupation

An equal number of subjects—40%—were in school or employed full time. Of those in school, all but 11% were working either part or full time. Only 30 subjects (15%) were neither employed nor in school and 6 of these were full time housewives.

All but 25% of the subjects had completed high school and a few of the youngest subjects were currently in high school. Twelve subjects were college graduates and 2 held masters degrees. Seventy-two subjects (36%) had some college education and some of them were currently attending college. Fifty-five percent of the subjects had been average or C students in their most recent school experience, 26% had received above average grades, and 19% had received below average or failing grades.

As might be expected, employment and school enrollment were significantly related to age with a majority (65%) of those aged 17 to 20 in school and only 8% of the 23-to 26-year-olds in school. Similarly, the age group having the most subjects (69%) who were employed part or full time was the 23-28 year old group, followed by a 60% employment rate in the 21-22 year old group (X^2 = 55.43, p< .0001). A somewhat unexpected finding was that the oldest age group also had the most subjects (22%) who were neither employed nor in school.

Employment histories showed that a majority (65%) of the subjects had never been fired from a job. Of the 32% who had been fired, the most frequent reasons were difficulty with a boss (35%) and difficulty meeting job requirements (15%).

There were also significant differences between males and females in relation to employment and school (X^2 = 16.75, 6 df, p <.01). More males (47%) than females (21%) were employed full time while more females (66%) than males (37%) were in school. This difference could not be related to age since there were no significant differences in age distribution of males and females.

Subjects' occupations ranged from unskilled to professional with 42% holding lesser white collar jobs. This concentration of subjects in the lesser white collar category was partly attributed to the student status of 54 subjects. Removal of students from this category leaves 14% of the subjects in lesser white collar positions. Eight percent of the subjects were in professional or semi-professional occupations, 29% skilled or semiskilled, and 18% in unskilled occupations. Sixteen subjects had been in military service and an additional 10 subjects were in service when interviewed.

Living Arrangements

Of the subjects, 53% were living with their parents, 23% with spouses, 15% with siblings and roomates, and 8% alone. Subjects' living arrangements were related to age with 79% of the 17 to 20 year olds living with their parents and 46% of the 23 to 28 year olds living with their spouses (X^2 = 58.52, p<.0001). There was no significant difference between males and females in their living arrangements although 13 men and only one woman lived alone.

Most (80%) of the subjects had changed their place of residence at least once in the past 10 years and 53% had made more than one move. Changes were related to family moves, and to the subjects' separation from their parents to go to college, to marry, or to live independently. There was relatively little geographic mobility in the sample. Seventy-four percent of the subjects still lived in the greater St. Louis area, 10% in other parts of Missouri, and 16% in other states. The 32 subjects interviewed outside of Missouri were in all regions of the United States.

Health

Subjects were generally in satisfactory health with 40% reporting that their health was average, 58% excellent, and 1.5% poor. However, more than half (61%) had been hospitalized in the past 10 years, with 50% hospitalized for physical illness or an accident and 11% hospitalized for psychiatric illness. There was no significant sex difference in the psychiatric hospitalizations. At least 11 subjects had attempted suicide. Moreover, this number is probably low since fewer than half the subjects were asked specifically about suicide.

Drug and Alcohol Use

The incidence of drug and alcohol use was based on subjects' self reports. Fifty-seven percent stated that they had never used drugs and 74% said that they were not using drugs at the time of follow-up. Marijuana was used by 25% of the subjects and 17% used other drugs. Frequency of drug use was daily for 8% of the 200 subjects, weekly for 12%, and rarely for 21%. Drug and alcohol use were significantly related to sex, with more males than females utilizing drugs ($X^2 = 14.73$, 4 df, p<.005) and alcohol ($X^2 = 17.47$, 3 df, p<.006).

More subjects used alcohol than drugs, although the frequency of alcohol use was not high. Of the subjects, 47.5% drank occasionally, 15% about once a week, 7.6% several times a week, and 15 subjects (7.6%) reported daily drinking.

Law Violations

Sixty-seven subjects (32%) reported law violations other than traffic citations. However, 29 of these subjects (14%) stated that they had not been arrested or jailed. Nineteen percent (38 subjects) had been arrested and half of them (17 subjects) had been jailed. Most offenses were misdemeanors, although 8 subjects had been cited for felonies. Law violations included several teenage runaways and subsequent placement in juvenile detention centers, as well as adult offenses. Law violations were sex related with 3 females and 64 males involved in some type of law violation ($X^2 = 21.40$, 4 df, p < .003).

In summary, the typical subject was a 21-year-old white, single, male high school graduate who was currently employed in a skilled, semi-skilled, or unskilled occupation and/or was enrolled in school. He was living with parents or spouse in the greater St. Louis area, but had changed residence at least once in recent years. He was in good health, did not abuse drugs, and drank in moderation.

Assessment of Social Functioning

A measure of adult social functioning was derived by summing the ratings on the five social adjustment items and thereby obtaining a score called Adult Sum of Social Adjustment (ASSA). The mean of the ASSA rating was 11.28 with a range of 5 to 23. Subjects' overall Adult Life Adjustment Ratings (ALAR) were made on a 5-point scale (Item F of Social Adjustment Scale in Appendix B). Reliability of these ratings was assessed through having two of the research staff interview a subject together and make their ratings independently. Interjudge coefficients of correlation ranged from .408 for the 5 SA items and .515 for the overall ALAR ratings (Appendix C).

As seen in Table 8; 53.5% of the subjects were rated as functioning well or with mild problems (rated 1 or 2), while 27.5% showed moderate distrubance in functioning (rated 3), and 19% were rated as severely maladjusted (4 and 5). Table 8 also shows the frequencies of each level of adjustment for these subjects in childhood. The mean rating was 3.32 in childhood and 2.46 in adulthood.

Subjects rated severely maladjusted were usually unemployed and not in school, were likely to have had psychiatric hospitalizations and had serious difficulties in interpersonal relationships. In contrast, those rated as healthy or with mild problems were functioning well in their jobs or school, and had constructive interpersonal relationships. There were no significant differences in social adjustment ratings for males and females nor for different age groups.

Table 8.　Global Life Adjustment Ratings

Rating	Childhood[a]		Follow-up[b]	
	N = 200	%	N = 200	%
1	0	0	43	21.5
2	11	5.5	64	32.0
3	115	57.5	55	27.5
4	73	36.5	34	17.0
5	1	.5	4	2.0

[a]Mean = 3.32; SD = .58.
[b]Mean = 2.46; SD = 1.07.

In five different areas of social functioning subjects were rated healthiest in the areas which required the least intense interpersonal relationships—school or work and larger society—and they were rated slightly less healthy in more intense areas, that is, relationships with their families and with peers. The means for the different social functioning areas are presented below.

Relationships with teachers or employers	2.0
Work or school performance	2.2
Functioning in society	2.2
Relationships with family	2.3
Relationships with peers	2.4

In summary, slightly more than half of the subjects were rated as functioning quite adequately in adulthood, about one fourth showed considerable difficulty in social functioning, and one fifth had major problems which prevented them from leading constructive, stable lives.

Relationship Between Childhood Variables and Assessment of Adult Adjustment

The major hypothesis of this study was that overall social and personal adjustment of young adults who were seen at the Clinic could be predicted from early behavioral, social, symptomatic, and clinical data. It will be recalled that the various ratings of childhood data (Table 7) correlated significantly.

This hypothesis was tested by analyzing the relationships between child- hood variables and ratings of adult social adjustment (ASSA). As will be recalled, ASSA is a rating of social adjustment at follow-up derived from summing the ratings in five different areas of social functioning. Two types of analyses were carried out: Pearson r correlations between specific childhood data and ASSA; and two-way ANOVA of childhood variables and sex with ASSA as the dependent variable.

The data provide some support for the hypothesis although the correlations are hardly high enough to be predictive.

As evident in Table 9, CSSA had the highest correlation with adult social adjustment ratings, while CLAR correlated less well but also significantly. Parents' socioeconomic status was also significantly related to adult outcome. Two types of childhood clinical data were significantly correlated with ASSA: intensity of disturbance as judged and recorded during the diagnostic conference and the Full Scale Intelligence Quotient. The FSIQ correlation is negative, indicating that greater maladjustment was associated with lower IQ. The sum of disturbance ratings based on psychological test data and those

Table 9.   Correlations Between Major Childhood Variables and Ratings of Adult Functioning (ASSA)

Childhood Variables	Correlations with ASSA[a]	
Childhood sum SA: CSSA	.2231	$p < .001$
Intensity of disturbance	.1999	$p < .010$
Full scale IQ	-.1775	$p < .006$
SES	.1584	$p < .013$
Child life adjustment rating: CLAR	.1414	$p < .023$
Total school behavior	.1367	$p < .031$
Sum weighted symptoms	.1198	$p < .060$
Psychiatric sum of disturbance	.1176	$p < .058$
Number of symptoms	.1055	n.s.
Psychological sum of disturbance	.0626	n.s.

[a]Pearson r.

ratings based on psychiatric interview data were not significantly related to adult functioning (significance level greater than .05), although the psychiatric rating showed a trend toward significance.

The number and severity of symptoms and problem behaviors reported by parents were not related to adult outcome at the .05 level of significance. However, school teacher reports of the number of symptomatic behaviors checked on a list of 29 items were significantly related to outcome.

Of the five individual life functioning areas which were assessed in both childhood and adulthood and summed to obtain the CSSA and ASSA ratings, four showed significant but modest correlations ranging from .12 to .23. These were family relationships, school or job functioning, relationships with teachers or bosses, and functioning in society. The fifth area, peer relationships, did not show a significant correlation between child and adult ratings.

It is evident from these findings that while there is, indeed, some relationship between adult outcome and the assessments of disturbance and maladjustment which brought these 200 children to child guidance, the correlations are not of a magnitude to allow for prediction. Inspection of the central tendencies and standard deviations of the child and adult social adjustment ratings may cast light on the reason for the modest correlation between the ratings of child and adult social adjustment.

As children, these 200 subjects had a mean social adjustment rating of 16.06 and as adults the mean was 11.28 on a scale of 5 to 25 points. The small standard deviation in the childhood ratings shows a concentration of subjects close to the mean, while the adult ratings show greater variation. The lower mean in adulthood indicates a general shift toward healthier functioning ratings for these subjects as adults in contrast to their childhood ratings (Table 10).

Table 10.   Child and Adult Social Adjustment

Adjustment	Mean	Standard Deviation
CSSA	16.06	1.96
ASSA	11.28	4.46

A different measure, the global ratings of life adjustment (CLAR), indicated even more clearly the concentration of child subjects in the moderate and severely disturbed categories, while the adults were distributed on all five points of the social adjustment scale (see Table 8). Of the child subjects, 94% were rated at points 3 and 4, 5.5% at point 2, and none was rated at point 1 (good adjustment). In contrast, 54% of the adults were rated at point 1 or 2 and 46% at points 3, 4, and 5, indicating considerably more variation in adult than in child ratings. Changes in global social adjustment ratings between childhood and adulthood were computed by subtracting the CLAR from the ALAR. Of the subjects, 63.5% obtained healthier ratings at follow-up, 23.5% retained the same rating, and 13% obtained ratings of greater maladjustment in adulthood than in childhood. Thus, social adjustment ratings made at 2 points in time show that a majority of the subjects improved their adjustment ratings over time, some stayed the same, and a small number (26) deteriorated in social adjustment ratings. There is some question about the validity of assessing change over time because of the differences in social adjustment behaviors at different developmental levels. Also, although many subjects' ratings improved, at least 9% of those rated as improved still showed moderate to severe maladjustment in their functioning.

Although correlations were modest, an effort was made to determine if a combination of childhood variables would be predictive of adult adjustment. A multiple regression analysis, using 41 childhood variables, was carried out. Only one variable, the CSSA rating, was predictive in this analysis, and addition of other variables did not strengthen the predictive power.

The second objective of the research was to determine which of the specific behavioral, social, and personality variables of childhood were associated with the degree of maladjustment in adult social functioning. Two-way analyses of variance of adult social adjustment ratings by the child's sex and other childhood variables produced some significant relationships.

Clinical Data

The clinical diagnosis made at the diagnostic conference in childhood significantly related to ratings of adult social adjustment ($F = 2.506$, 6/194 df, $p < 025$). As evident in Table 11, this relationship is due mainly to the much lower (good adjustment) adult ratings of the children with transient reactions

Table 11.   Childhood Diagnosis and Social Adjustment in Childhood and Adulthood

| | Social Adjustment | | |
Diagnosis	N = 195[a]	Mean CSSA	Mean ASSA
Transient reaction and developmental problems	10	14.45	7.60
Neurotic reaction	100	15.70	11.05
Neurotic behavior disorder	24	16.58	11.13
Character disorder	30	16.63	12.13
Borderline psychosis	15	18.06	13.67
Psychosis	4	17.00	9.75
Mental deficiency and brain syndrome	12	15.57	12.25

[a]Those categories containing a total of 5 subjects not included because of small numbers.

or developmental problems, neurotic reactions, and neurotic behavior disorders, compared with the higher (poor adjustment) adult ratings of the children diagnosed as character disorders and borderline psychotic. Sex was not a significant variable in this analysis. Since the number of children diagnosed as psychotic, retarded, or brain syndrome was so small (16), the data were re-analyzed with these subjects eliminated from the analysis: then ASSA was highly related to the diagnostic conference diagnosis (F = 3.662, 4/174 df, p < .007).

A research psychologist and psychiatrist, working independently, rated each child's clinical protocols on the same 12 personality characteristics, and on overall severity of disturbance. The 12 individual items contained in both the psychological and psychiatric ratings were analyzed. Two psychological items were significant: concreteness (F = 2.471, 1/199 df, p<.05) and efficiency of defenses (F = 3.271, 3/199 df, p< .007). However, neither item showed a linear relationship although the most severe disturbance rating in each was indicative of the most severe impairment in adult social functioning.

Several of the psychological and psychiatric items showed a sex-linked interaction in relation to adult adjustment ratings. These included the psychological severity of disturbance and degree of identity disturbance. For females the psychological severity of disturbance rating was significantly related to adult adjustment ratings, but not in a meaningful way since the least and most disturbed ratings were related to poor adult social adjustment. For males the type of anxiety, rated by psychiatrists, was significant (F = 3.287, 2/104 df, p <.04). Internal anxiety manifested by boys was related to good adult ratings and external anxiety to poor adult ratings. Comparison of disturbance in identity showed a sex difference. Males with poor ratings in identity had poor adult ratings and girls with poor identity ratings had positive adult social adjustment ratings (t = 3.77, 62 df, p < .001).

Several developmental items showed significant differences between males and females with the differences indicating opposite effects on adult social adjustment ratings. Low birth weight (t = 2.57, 15.90 df, p<.021) and less than full-term pregnancy (t = 2.90, 17.70 df, p<.010) were related to poor outcome ratings for males and healthy adult ratings for females.

Those children who were breast fed had better adult ratings than those who were not, but of those who were breast fed, absence of problems in feeding was related to poor adult ratings and the presence of 1 or 2 problems with breast feeding was related to positive adult adjustment ratings (F = 3.35, 4/195 df, p<.011).

Application Data

Information about the child's problems, reasons for referral, and various aspects of his family situation were analyzed by a two-way ANOVA design. A variety of problems brought the subjects to the clinic in childhood. Two of these problems had opposite relationships to adult functioning for males and females. Behavior problems in the home (t = 3.27, 32.83 df, p<.003) and behavior problems outside the home (t = 5.02, 20.43, df, p<.001) were related to poor adult ratings for males and good ratings for females.

There was a linear relationship between the age at which a child's problems were first noticed and his adult ratings (F = 3.154, 6/194 df, p<.009), in that the younger children had poorer adult adjustment ratings. However, children were not brought to the Clinic when their problems were first noticed. The child's age at time of clinic application showed some relationship to adult functioning in that two groups of children, those 5 and 6 and those 11 and 12 years of age had poorer adult ratings than other age groups (F = 1.78, 9/199 df, p<.07).

First born children had significantly better adult adjustment ratings than those who were born later, with a progressive decline in adult ratings as birth order increased through the fourth child (F = 3.176, 4/197 df, p<.015).

Family factors related to the subjects' adult social adjustment ratings include parents' education, social class, father's hours of employment, and religion. The parents' socioeconomic status is weakly but significantly correlated with the subjects' adult adjustment ratings (r = .1584, p<.013). The parents' education and occupation were used to compute SES, but only parents' educational level by itself is related to subjects' adult functioning. Although there is not a fully linear relationship between father's education and subjects' adult functioning, those subjects who came from families with fathers having more than a high school education or less than 6th grade education had the best ratings, while those whose fathers had completed 7th, 8th, or 9th grades had less adequate ratings (F = 2.587, 7/178 df, p<.02). The relationship of mothers' education to subjects' adult functioning ratings was not as strong but followed a linear pattern with higher education related to better adult ratings (F = 2.27, 4/193 df, p < .062).

The religion of subjects and their mothers was significantly related to adult ratings for male subjects but not for female subjects. For males, Jewish subjects had the best adult ratings, followed by Protestants, and Catholics had the poorest ratings (F = 2.894, 2/130 df, p<.057). The same pattern was evident in analyzing mothers' religion, although the relationship was considerably stronger than that of child's religion (F = 5.26, 2/135 df, p<.006). Boys' and girls' religion was compared. There were no significant sex differences for the three religious groups. However, comparison of mothers' religion by child's sex shows that having a Catholic mother is related to positive adult ratings for girls and negative adult ratings for boys (t = 3.0, 49 df, p<.004).

Parental Characteristics

Parents were rated on 14 factors that were descriptive of their functioning, their attitudes toward their children, and their interaction with them. The items included ratings of each parent's emotional stability, coping capacity, parents' relationship to each other, their feelings about the pregnancy and the child, and their reactions to the child's problems. None of these items was related to subjects' adult functioning ratings.

School Behaviors

Additional analyses of school behaviors were carried out by Janes and Hesselbrock (1978) to determine if specific child behaviors reported by teachers as well as the total number of behaviors present were predictive of adult social functioning. A 2 X 2 ANOVA design was used to determine the predictive significance of each item by sex. For boys and girls combined, three items were associated with poor adult functioning: "fails to get along with other children" (F = 8.900, 1/186 df, p<.005), "temper display" (F = 5.712, 1/186 df, p<.02), and "selfish" (F = 4.68, 1/186 df, p<.05).

Sex differences were evident in several items. For boys, items related to poor adult social adjustment ratings were "fails to get along with other children" (t = 2.68, 135 df, p<.005), "selfish" (t = 2.49, 135 df, p<.02), "fights" (t = 1.88, 135 df, p<.10), and "prefers younger children" (t = 1.85, 135 df, p<.10). For girls, the items associated most with poor adult social functioning ratings were "withdrawn" (t = 3.08, 48 df, p<.005), "temper display" (t = 2.85, 48 df, p<.005), and "fails to get along with other children" (t = 1.33, 48 df, p<.10).

The number of school behavior items checked as well as three items for the group as a whole were related to adult social adjustment ratings. Specific items of significance differed for boys and girls except for the item "failure to get along with other children," which was highly significant for boys and showed a trend toward significance for girls.

Symptoms

Two-way ANOVA tests of a 38-item symptom list from childhood showed three symptoms to be significantly related to adult adjustment ratings for the total group, and an additional four symptoms had significant sex interaction effects. The symptoms related to poor adult adjustment were learning problems (F = 4.256, p < .01), reaction to change (F = 3.62, p < .02), and respiratory problems (F = 2.71, p < .05). Those symptoms showing a sex interaction effect were bowel control problems (F = 3.36, p < .04), school absence (F = 2.46, p < .01), unusual fears (F = 2.77, p < .03), and accident proneness (F = 3.19, p < .05). However, when these symptoms were further analyzed by sex, that is, for boys, for girls, and comparing boys and girls, only one symptom was related to adult adjustment. For boys but not for girls, the symptom of accident proneness was significantly related to adult functioning ratings. The ratings on this symptom were dichotomized so that differences are based on presence or absence of the symptom (t = -2.76, 139 df, p < .007). No other sex differences were found.

Mothers were asked, at follow-up interview, to check a symptom list as they saw their son or daughter at present and mail it to the interviewer. The son or daughter was also asked to fill out the list about himself independently.

Eighty-five (42.5%) of the subjects and 71 (35.5%) of the mothers returned the completed forms. Included in these returns were 51 pairs of lists in which both the young adult and mother complied. There was a correlation of .488 (Pearson r, p < .001) between the number of symptoms checked by mothers and subjects and an r of .605 (p < .001) between the sums of weighted symptoms (specifying intensity of each symptom).

The returns from the mothers could also be compared to the equivalent symptom lists they had filled out on their children at the time of their original Clinic contacts. The Pearson r between the 69 pairs of symptom lists available for both periods in time was .264 (p < .02) for the number of symptoms checked and .305 (p < .01) for the sums of weighted symptoms. These correlations indicate significant relationships between current perceptions of the young adults by the mother and self, and also between mothers' perception of him or her now and in childhood. The correlations are based on only 25.5 to 34.5% of the total research sample of 200 mother-subject pairs, however, and the extent of bias in the composition of the subsample is not known.

Relationship of Young Adult Pathology
and Selected Childhood Variables

At follow-up two groups of subjects reported behavior that was considered pathological. These groups were composed of subjects who had experienced psychiatric hospitalization in late adolescence or early adulthood, and those whose antisocial behavior had led to law violations. Those subjects (21) who had been in psychiatric hospitals were compared with those who reported no hospitalization; and those subjects (38) who reported law violations were compared with those who reported that they had not had any law violations

Law violators differed from non-law violators in adult social adjustment ratings and on 4 of 14 childhood variables analyzed. Those who had experienced psychiatric hospitalization differed from those not hospitalized in adult social adjustment ratings and on 3 of 14 childhood variables. These differences are evident in Table 12.

Childhood variables that did not differentiate these groups included psychiatric and psychological sum of disturbance ratings, birth and pregnancy complications, symptoms, and IQ. As was true for the whole sample, indices of poor social adjustment were the most dependable predictors to deviance in adulthood, in this case law violation and hospitalization for psychiatric illness. Both of these groups were also rated at the diagnostic conference in childhood as more severely disturbed than the rest of the sample of 200. In addition, total school misbehaviors were related to adult law violation and social class of parents was lower for those hospitalized for psychiatric illness than for the total sample.

Analysis of Variables Related to Persistence of Pathology from Childhood to Young Adulthood

Continuity in personality development was a concept implicit in this study. Thus, it was hypothesized that pathology in childhood would persist into young adulthood. Although the social adjustment ratings for the total group showed a shift toward healthier functioning in adulthood than childhood, over half of the subjects retained their relative position on the health-disturbance social adjustment scale at the two time periods assessed: at clinic evaluation and at follow-up. Four groups were identified: A) those rated least disturbed at both time points, B) those rated most disturbed at both time points, C) those who changed from least to most disturbed, and D) those who changed in the opposite direction—most to least disturbed. The distribution of these groups is presented in Table 13.

Thus, there was some support for the hypothesis of continuity in that 53.5% of the subjects retained their same relative position in relation to health or disturbance and 46.5% showed change in one direction or the other at two different time points: childhood evaluation and adult follow-up. *The least disturbed were unlikely to change while the most disturbed were likely to change toward health.*

No-change Groups

In the two groups that showed continuity, a number of variables differentiated those who remained least disturbed from those who remained most disturbed. Those variables related to persistence of disturbance are presented in Table 14.

Table 12. Variables Differentiating Those Violating Law and Those Psychiatrically Hospitalized from Other Follow-up Subjects

Variable	Law Violators (N = 38)			Psychiatric Hospitalization (N = 21)		
	t	df	sig.	t	df	sig.
Adult social adjustment	5.44	197	.001	3.89	196	.001
Child social adjustment	2.60	197	.010	2.59	196	.010
Child life adjustment rating	2.50	197	.013	.52	196	n.s.
Intensity of disturbance	2.49	197	.014	2.48	190	.014
Total school behavior	1.90	184	.059	.95	183	n.s.
Psychological severity	.71	197	n.s.	.81	196	n.s.
Psychiatric severity	.10	179	n.s.	.04	178	n.s.
Total # symptoms	.10	197	n.s.	.68	196	n.s.
Birth complications	1.42	197	n.s.	.59	196	n.s.
Pregnancy complications	1.12	197	n.s.	.68	196	n.s.
Weighted symptoms	1.24	167	n.s.	.45	166	n.s.
Psychological disturbance	.14	197	n.s.	.39	196	n.s.
Psychiatric disturbance	.35	176	n.s.	.41	175	n.s.
SES	.36	197	n.s.	2.99	196	.003
FS IQ	.42	196	n.s.	.08	195	n.s.

Table 13.   Change in Social Adjustment Ratings from Time I (Child) to Time II (Follow-up)[a]

Change Groups	N	Percent
No change (Groups A and B)		
Least disturbed both times: $<$ Mean	70	35
Most disturbed both times: $>$ Mean	37	18.5
Change (Groups C and D)		
Least to most disturbed	43	21.5
Most to least disturbed	50	25

[a] $X^2 = 7.38$, $p < .01$.

Several early developmental factors differentiated these two groups. Those subjects who remained most disturbed as contrasted to those who remained minimally disturbed were more likely to be underweight at birth, and to show disturbed behavior in infancy; specifically, bed shaking and unusual emotional behavior.

Family environment differed significantly for these two groups. For the least disturbed group parents were likely to be living together (85%), the subject had not experienced a parental loss under 6 years of age (91%), grandparents had never lived in the home (82%), and their mothers came from small town or suburban areas (54%). In contrast, the most disturbed group had experienced loss of a parent before age 6 (35%), parental death, separation, or divorce (34%), grandparents in the home (35%), and had mothers who came from large cities (71%). In the no-change groups first born children fared better than later born with 80% of the first born in the least disturbed group and 20% in the most disturbed group.

The subjects who remained in the most disturbed group differed from the least disturbed group in a number of symptomatic behaviors, behaviors that tended to bring the child into negative interaction with others. As reported by parents, subjects in the most disturbed group were impulsive (92%), resistive (89%), related poorly to adults (77%), were accident prone (44%), were depressed, and tended to show antisocial behavior. Thus, the presence of these symptoms was greater in the consistently most disturbed than in the consistently least disturbed group.

Similarly, those subjects who continued to be disturbed at follow-up differed, as children, from those remaining least disturbed in more frequently showing the following school-reported behaviors: selfish (23%), disobedient (34%), temper outbursts (40%), lying (22%), fighting (31%), and poor relationships with other children. The most significant difference between the two groups was that of poor peer relationships, reported for over 60% of the most disturbed children and 20% of the least disturbed children. It was noted that the proportion of children showing symptomatic behaviors, as reported by teachers, was somewhat less than the proportion reported to have symptoms according to parents.

The types of behavior prevalent in the persistently "most disturbed" group were generally antisocial. In addition, this group tended to externalize anxiety, were more likely to show extreme emotionality, and were more often diagnosed as character disorders, borderline, or brain syndrome (55%); while those with least disturbance at both time points were diagnosed neurotic or showed transient or developmental difficulties (77%). On ratings of intensity of disturbance, 91% of the most disturbed in social adjustment and 49% of the least disturbed obtained clinical ratings of very intense disturbance (4 or 5 on a 5-point scale) in childhood.

Finally, the nonchanging "most disturbed" group had somewhat lower IQs than the nonchanging "least disturbed" group. Fifty percent of the latter had IQs of 110 or above while 70% of the former group had IQs under 110.

The two no-change groups did not differ significantly in age, sex, or socioeconomic status nor did treatment or the lack of it differentiate the two groups. Most of the ratings of parents' adjustment, coping, feelings about the child, discipline, and reaction to the child's problems showed significant differences between the two groups. However, since these items were based on the same data used to identify the subjects as most or least disturbed in childhood and were significantly correlated with child social adjustment ratings (r = .30 to .39), their importance seemed more related to the high intercorrelations of items in the measuring instrument than to meaningful differences between the two groups. This explanation applies to those items in the comparison of the two change groups as well as the two no-change groups.

Change Groups

In comparing the change groups, we found that for those who obtained healthier adult than child ratings and those who obtained poorer adult than child ratings, a few variables showed significant differences between the two groups (Table 14). However, fewer variables were significant in differentiating these two change groups than for the no-change groups, and most of the variables which proved to be significant were different from those differentiating the no-change groups. Subjects in the group which changed from disturbance to health, as contrasted to the group which changed to disturbance, more frequently showed symptoms of a neurotic type in childhood: compulsivity, restlessness, and extreme reaction to change. They also had poor peer relationships and heart difficulties. One school behavior was associated with positive change, that of resistant behavior.

Intensity of childhood disturbance was significantly greater for those children who changed toward health than for those who became more

Table 14. Variables Differentiating No-Change Group A from No-Change B and Those Differentiating Changed Group C from Changed Group D[a]

Variable	Group A vs. Group B		Group C vs. Group D	
	X^2	p	X^2	p
Pregnancy and early development				
Birth weight low	4.14	.05		
Bed shaking	4.91[b]	.027		
Unusual emotional behavior	7.29	.01		
Family situation				
No absence of parent for $\leq$ 6 months before age 6	10.11	.01		
Parents together	5.07	.05		
Grandparents never lived in home	13.44	.001		
Mother's home town not a large city	6.22	.05		
Less than two changes in residence			11.66	.001
First born	10.12	.01		
Presence of specific symptoms				
Depressed	11.43	.003		
Impulsive	4.90	.026		
Resistant	3.86	.049		
Antisocial	3.75	.053		
Accident prone	11.79	.001		
Poor relations with adults	4.29	.038		
Poor relations with peers			6.04	.014
Reaction to change			3.89	.048
Compulsive			8.57	.003
Restless			5.03	.025
Heart problems			9.69	.002

Table 14. Variables Differentiating No-Change Group A from No-Change B and Those Differentiating Changed Group C from Changed Group D[a] (Cont'd)

Variable	Group A vs. Group B		Group C vs. Group D	
	X^2	p	X^2	p
Presence of specific school behaviors				
Selfish	9.97	.001		
Disobedient	4.39	.036		
Temper	8.37	.003		
Lying	4.40	.036		
Poor social relations	14.09	.001		
Fights	7.65	.006		
Resistant			4.78	.029
Clinical data				
FS IQ	18.05^c	.004		
Diagnosis	9.70	.001		
Externalized anxiety	6.98^b	.031		
Emotionality	7.01^b	.05		
Severity of anxiety			9.00^b	.029
Object relations			8.44^c	.037
Intensity			10.46^c	.015
	22.81	.001	5.01	.025

[a]Group A: Social adjustment at or below mean in childhood and at follow-up (continuously least disturbed)

Group B: Social adjustment above mean in childhood and at follow-up (continuously most disturbed)

Group A had more positive position on differentiating variables than Group B.

Group C: Social adjustment below mean in childhood and above mean in adulthood (least to most disturbed)

Group D: Social adjustment above mean in childhood and below mean in adulthood (most to least disturbed)

Group D had more positive position on differentiating variables than Group C.

[b] = 2df

[c] = 3df, all others = 1df

disturbed. Extreme emotionality, severe anxiety, and impaired object relations were more frequent in the group which changed to health than in the group which obtained poorer adult than child ratings. The two groups which changed did not differ significantly in IQ or diagnosis.

Two variables that were significantly related to both change and lack of change were intensity of disturbance and emotionality. The children who were most disturbed in both childhood and adulthood on the social adjustment scale and those who were disturbed in childhood and less disturbed in adulthood had childhood clinical ratings of intense disturbance at the Clinic diagnostic conference.

In summary, over half of the subjects retained their relative position of disturbance or health in child and adult social adjustment ratings. The rest of the subjects showed change in either a positive or negative direction. A number of variables differentiated those who remained most disturbed from those who remained least disturbed. Those variables most frequently found in the disturbed group included early developmental difficulties, changes in family membership such as loss of parents or addition of grandparents to the family, symptoms of acting out as reported by parents and by teachers, low IQ, and psychiatric diagnosis. Fewer, but different, variables showed significant differences between those subjects who changed in a positive direction and those who changed in a negative direction. Age, sex, social class, and treatment were not significant in either change or no-change comparisons.

Relationship of Treatment to Adult Social Functioning

A third objective of the research was to determine the extent to which treatment reduced the persistence of pathology from childhood to adulthood.

The Clinic recommended treatment for 195 children and no treatment for four children. No recommendation was recorded for one child. Reterral to other agencies or private practitioners was recommended for 65 children, while Clinic treatment was recommended for 130. However, 35 families refused Clinic treatment: 11 refused at the time of the postdiagnostic conference and 24 refused after being on a waiting list. Reasons for refusal of Clinic treatment included disagreement with the recommendation, a desire to obtain immediate treatment rather than go onto a waiting list, and improvement in the child's difficulties between the diagnostic evaluation and the time Clinic treatment was offered.

Eighty-nine children were actually treated at the Clinic and parents of three other children were treated, although their children were not. Fifty-nine children obtained treatment outside the Clinic through social agencies or private practitioners. There were no significant differences in the childhood social adjustment ratings of those who accepted Clinic treatment or referral and those who refused Clinic treatment prior to or after being on the waiting list, or those who refused referral.

Treatment Provided and Adult Outcome

On the basis of Clinic records and self reports at follow-up it was possible to identify three treatment groups: those who had Clinic treatment, those who had Clinic treatment and later obtained additional treatment, those who had treatment outside the Clinic, sometime between Clinic evaluation and follow-up. A fourth group reported no treatment following Clinic evaluation. The differences between these four groups in ratings of childhood social adjustment only approached significance (F = 2.54, p < .106), but they showed highly significant differences in adult adjustment (F = 12.32, 3/196df, p < .001). The four groups and the mean child and adult social functioning ratings of each group are presented in Table 15.

It is evident that those subjects who had no treatment obtained much healthier ASSA ratings than those who received treatment of some kind. However, the Clinic treated group obtained a mean ASSA rating (10.67) somewhat healthier than the mean for the total sample (11.28).

Consistent data regarding treatment were not collected for those subjects who obtained treatment subsequent to their Clinic evaluations or to their Clinic treatment. The duration and type of treatment were not known, for all the subjects, nor the age at which it was obtained. Some subjects reported meaningful treatment of several years duration, some recalled going to a social agency or therapist but could not remember when or for how long, others reported brief treatment during adolescence or early adulthood, and 21 subjects reported one or more periods of psychiatric hospitalization occurring as early as age 11 up through age 23. Thus, there was wide variation in the nature and extent of subjects' treatment experiences outside the Clinic. Because of the lack of specific information about these treatment experiences outside the Clinic it was not possible to assess their effects.

However, information about some treatment variables was available for those subjects who received Clinic treatment and they were compared with

Table 15. Mean Sum of Child and Adult Social Adjustment Ratings

Groups	N	Child SSA	Adult SSA
Clinic treatment	54	15.87	10.67
Other treatment	59	16.47	12.95
Clinic and other treatment	35	16.28	13.23
No treatment	52	15.63	8.83
Total	200	16.06	11.28

those subjects who reported no treatment experience. Although these two groups did not meet the criterion of random assignment for an experimental design, they did appear comparable in many ways.

The untreated group (N = 52), composed of those subjects who reported no treatment following Clinic evaluation, obtained significantly healthier adult adjustment ratings than the treated group (N = 54) composed of those subjects who were treated at the Clinic and received no subsequent treatment. The two groups were compared on two items: ALAR (t = 2.23, 104 df, p < .028) and ASSA (t = 3.03, 99.72 df, p < .003) Although significantly different on adult ratings, both groups showed a high proportion of subjects with healthier adult global (life) adjustment ratings than child ratings: 7€% of those treated and 82.7% of those not treated.

Comparison of Clinic-treated with Untreated Groups on Childhood Variables

There were no significant differences between the two groups in age at time of Clinic evaluation, age at follow-up, sex, FSIQ, parents' socioeconomic status, and parents' education.

The two groups were not significantly different in most childhood ratings of disturbance, diagnosis, symptomatic behaviors, early development and early trauma. Items analyzed and tests used to determine comparability of the two groups are contained in Table 16.

Thus, it is possible but unlikely that the treated group was slightly more disturbed in childhood than the untreated group; on all but one of the 17 childhood variables tested there were no statistically significant differences between the groups.

Family environmental factors were examined to determine the comparability of the two groups. No significant differences were found in parents' marital status, mother's employment, child's birth order, or in ratings of parents' emotional stability, coping capacities, marital relationships, or reaction to the child's problems.

In summary, subjects who received no treatment obtained significantly healthier ratings of adult social functioning than those who had Clinic treatment. The groups were comparable in age, sex, IQ, and socioeconomic status. There were no significant differences in family environment and parental functioning. The groups did not differ significantly in psychiatric diagnosis or in degree of disturbance in childhood with the exception of a weak difference on one rating (psychiatric severity of disturbance). The only major difference between the groups was that one group of parents chose to follow the Clinic recommendation for treatment, whereas the other group of parents did not follow the recommendation. Thus, self-selection led families into or away from treatment. The meaning of this selection is not known.

Table 16.   Comparison of Treated and Untreated Groups on Childhood Variables

| | Mean | |
Childhood Variable	Treated	Untreated
Sum of social adjustment	15.87	15.63
Life adjustment rating	3.35	3.29
Sum of psychiatric disturbance	31.06	29.23
Sum of psychological disturbance	35.46	35.09
Severity of disturbance-psychiatric[a]	3.08	2.80
Severity of disturbance-psychological	3.77	3.15
Intensity of disturbance	3.94	3.69
Number of symptoms	17.07	18.00
Number of school behaviors	4.18	4.77
Pregnancy complications	.98	1.31
Birth complications	1.93	1.77
Accidents	.86	.76
Illnesses	2.57	2.86
Operations	1.34	1.27
Diagnosis[c]		
Birth weight[c]		
Antisocial behavior[b]		

[a] $t = 1.84$, 94 df, $p < .069$; difference between all other means n.s.
[b] $X^2 = 5.54$, $p < .018$.
[c] Diagnosis and birth weight n.s.

Analysis of Treatment Variables in the Clinic-Treated Group

The length of treatment, type of treatment, number of therapists, the therapist's status as staff member or trainee (psychiatric fellow, psychology intern, or social work student) and subject's recall of the helpfulness of Clinic treatment were analyzed in relation to ASSA for the Clinic treated group.

The length of treatment varied from one month to over three years. There was a trend toward a significant relationship between length of treatment and ASSA with those children who were in treatment more than two years, as contrasted to those receiving shorter treatment, obtaining the healthiest ASSA ratings ($F = 2.84$, 2/49, $p. < .092$). However, the length of parental treatment was not related to subjects' ASSA. The length of treatment is presented in Table 17.

The type of treatment received by children and parents was not related to ASSA. The predominant child treatment was individual therapy (29) with 24 children receiving family or group treatment or a combination of individual, family, and group. The type of treatment was not known for one subject. Parents were treated mainly through joint interviews or a combination of individual and joint (21), although family, group, or some combination were

Table 17.   Length of Treatment of Child, Mother, Father

Duration	Child N = 54	Mother N = 53	Father N = 42
Less than 1 year	18	26	20
1-2 years	20	13	12
More than 2 years	14	12	9
Unknown	2	2	1

used with 21 mothers and 17 fathers, and individual treatment was provided for 9 mothers and 3 fathers. Fifty-three mothers were involved in treatment and 42 fathers. There was no relationship between ASSA and the involvement of one or both parents in treatment.

The majority of children and parents were treated by one therapist, although 12 children, 12 mothers, and 10 fathers had more than one therapist. The number of therapists for parents was not related to ASSA, but children who had more than one therapist had slightly better ASSA ratings than those with only one therapist ($t = 1.84$, 51 df, $p < .071$). Those children with more than one therapist remained in treatment significantly longer than those with only one therapist ($F = 11.38$, $1/49$ df, $p < .042$). However, an analysis of covariance of number of therapists and length of treatment with ASSA as the dependent variable proved this relationship to be nonsignificant.

Children treated by staff members or by both a staff member and a trainee had significantly better ASSA ratings ($F = 3.34$, $2/50$ df, $p < .042$) than those treated by trainees alone. This difference was not evident for parents. There was no significant difference in the child's intensity of disturbance rating for the different categories of therapists. The majority of children and parents were treated by staff members, as is evident in Table 18.

The child's diagnosis was not related to ASSA, nor did the diagnosis of those treated differ significantly from the diagnosis of the total sample. The diagnostic categories of the treated group are shown in Table 19.

At follow-up, subjects and mothers were asked to assess the helpfulness of Clinic treatment. Thirty-five former child patients recalled their treatment experience. Eighteen subjects considered it helpful and 17 indicated it was not

Table 18.   Status of Clinic Therapist for Child, Mother, Father

Status of Therapist	Child N = 53	Mother N = 53	Father N = 42
Staff member	29	35	27
Trainee	17	6	5
Both staff and trainee	7	12	10

helpful. Mothers were somewhat more positive with 33 recalling the experience as helpful and 12 stating it was not helpful. The factor of helpfulness was not related to ASSA. It was noted that there was considerable missing data on this item, partly because of subjects' lack of recall of the experience or feeling that they could not evaluate it.

In summary, children treated by staff members as contrasted to trainees obtained significantly healthier adult adjustment ratings. There was a trend toward healthier adult ratings as the length of treatment increased. The type of treatment, the intensity of the child's disturbance, and clinical diagnosis were not related to adult adjustment ratings. Those children who received treatment obtained significantly poorer ASSA ratings than those children not treated although the mean ASSA ratings of both the treated and nontreated groups were improved over the mean childhood social adjustment rating of the total sample.

Table 19. Diagnoses of Treated Children and of Total Sample

Diagnostic Category	Clinic Treatment N = 54	%	Total Group N = 200	' %
Developmental or transient disorder	2	3.7	11	5.5
Neurotic reaction	28	51.9	100	51.0
Neurotic behavior disorder	9	16.7	24	12.0
Character disorder	6	11.1	30	15.0
Borderline psychosis	6	11.1	15	7.5
Other	3	5.5	20	10.0

CHAPTER 5

Summary and Discussion of Findings

The findings of this study agree in general with those of most of the other carefully done follow-up studies reported in the literature and reviewed in the Kohlberg et al. (1972), Robins (1972), Lewis (1965) and Levitt (1971) articles. Briefly stated, they are:

1. Except for extreme personality deviations, that is, psychoses and extreme antisocial behavior, there seems to be little continuity between child and adult disturbances.

2. The diagnosis of neurosis in childhood, a diagnosis which often encompasses a large proportion of child guidance referrals and those taken into treatment, does not portend severe maladjustment in adulthood. Half of the 200 children in this research sample were diagnosed as neurotic at their clinic diagnostic conference and their adult social adjustment was rated at an average significantly better than those diagnosed character disorders or borderline psychotic. These findings agree with most recent research.

3. Most children referred to child guidance can be expected to improve in adjustment into adulthood with or without therapy. Yet, a sizeable proportion of referrals will be moderately to severely disturbed in adulthood. These two categories comprised 46% of the subjects in the present research and in these there was a high incidence of psychiatric hospitalization and law violation.

4. Children at the healthier end of the adjustment continuum are likely to remain relatively healthy in adulthood while children with severe problems in childhood may remain disturbed *or* improve. Of the subjects, 63.5% obtained healthier ratings in this follow-up: 23.5% retained the same rating, and only 13% were rated more maladjusted in adulthood than in childhood. It is easier, as has been found by other researchers, to predict from (relative) health to health than it is from childhood disturbance to either health or maladjustment.

5. A few major childhood variables significantly differentiated those destined for poor adjustment in adulthood. Social adjustment in childhood as rated from data obtained from parental interviews and from written parental and school reports was the most powerful of

these variables. The rating of intensity of disturbance made at a diagnostic staff conference, social class, and IQ were also significantly related to degree of adult maladjustment.

6. A few specific childhood variables showed statistical significance for adult adjustment for the whole sample although the correlations were weak. These included the age at which the problems were first noticed (the younger the age the poorer the adult adjustment), being first born (related to better outcome), the total number of and a few specific school behaviors, especially failure to get along with other children, and a few symptoms such as learning problems and resistance to change.

7. When children who remained most disturbed were compared to those who remained least disturbed in adulthood, several variables differentiated the groups, including early developmental difficulties, change in family membership, symptoms of acting out, IQ, and psychiatric diagnosis.

8. As reported repeatedly in the literature, the sex of the child is an important consideration in identification of childhood variables that relate to outcome. Examples of such sex-related variables in the present research are two of the reasons for referral: behavior problems in the home and outside the home were related to poor adult ratings for males and *good* ratings for females. As is true in several other research reports, withdrawn behavior in girls related to poor outcome while more aggressive antisocial behavior related to later poor adjustment in boys.

9. One of the most important findings of this research is probably that of the significance of age in any attempt to predict outcome. Because of the changes associated with successive stages in the development of personality, the age at initial evaluation may be the crucial factor in predicting adult outcome. The present research agrees with several longitudinal studies that stress the importance of problems in the pre- or early adolescent period, about age 11 to 12, as foreshadowing later maladjustment. In addition, children whose problems press for attention early in life (before age 5) had poor outcomes.

10. The findings of this study relating therapy to outcome add to the accumulating evidence from other studies that children who receive outpatient therapy do not show better *social* adjustment at follow-up than children with similar diagnoses and judged to be equally disturbed who do not receive therapy. In the present study, psychotherapy was recommended for practically *all* the children in the sample of 200, and groups composed of those who actually went into

treatment at the clinic could be compared with those who, for one reason or another, failed to do so. The children without therapy received significantly better social adjustment ratings in adulthood than those who received clinic treatment. The meaning of these findings must be qualified by the fact that therapist and therapy variables were not controlled; by the limited nature (social adjustment) of the follow-up assessment, and by the possibility that the parents who refused treatment for their children may be a select group, for example, those who have relatively adequate coping capacities and/or who may have received sufficient help from the extended diagnostic process itself.

THE BASIC PROBLEM IN CLINICAL PREDICTION

This research project had the advantages of a sample of children with a variety of problems and a full and multi-level diagnostic assessment from which to forecast adult adjustment. The data were nearly uniform across subjects and could be quantified and analyzed statistically. Follow-up interviews with the 200 clinic children and their mothers were done in person and the evaluations were "blind," that is, without knowledge of the childhood findings. With all this richness and uniformity of childhood data and the careful, prospective planning for the follow-up, the results of the research are not as plentiful nor as definitive as was expected, and they, like those of many other follow-up studies reported in the literature, present the vagaries and complexities of human personality development rather than a blueprint of adjustment patterns from childhood to adulthood.

One core problem in the task of prediction is the difficulty of presenting in any statistical way the individual as a unit with all his assets and liabilities, each weighted for its importance to the gestalt. The weighing of each factor itself differs according to the nature of the rest of the factors both within the individual's own dynamics and within his family and broader environment. As yet, such complex profiles are not handled satisfactorily by statistical methods.

A research group at the Menninger Foundation (Sargent et al., 1968), convinced that prediction is meaningful only when based on the study of each person in all his complexity and set within his particular life context, began, in 1954, a long-term project to predict outcome of adult patients diagnosed and treated in long-term psychoanalytic psychotherapy. This project is a model of thorough consideration of the individual within an explicit, repeatable method of making predictions exclusively for him based on theory (psychoanalysis).

The Menninger researchers cast their predictions in an "if/then/because" formula. Their purpose was "to test these *clinical* predictions about treatment, made in advance of treatment, on which assignments to varying treatment modalities are based, and to use the predictive data for the better understanding of how empirical conditions, theoretical assumptions, and treatment consequences are specifically linked" (p. 27). The design in the Menninger research allowed for repeated observation over the years the patients were in clinic service and again two years after termination. The reports of the research include detailed analyses of the clinical prediction process.

The Menninger research, like that of the Hampstead Clinic (A. Freud, 1977), represents an ideal in terms of individualized prediction which, because of the effort, expense, and specialized setting required, is not likely to be a practical model. In our research, clinicians made an effort to take the whole person into account in their ratings but the follow-up was limited to one reassessment and the clinicians' global impression is recorded and treated in the analysis of data only as a diagnostic term or a rating of severity. While these two kinds of "distillate" variables can be expected to have some predictive value, they can in no way represent fully the complex interrelationship of variables within one individual and his milieu. A discursive account of each person's idioverse would do more justice to its complexity, but such an account could not be used statistically without separating out its component parts and reducing it, as were all the data, to treatment of specific variables through group statistics.

This problem was discussed by Rosenzweig (1958) and, more recently, in an article in the *American Psychologist* by Marceil (1977) who points out that two issues are involved in the controversy between "idiography" and "nomothesis," that is, the issues of theory *and* method. He points out that *either* of the two basic positions in theory, that man is more similar to than different from his fellow beings or that man is more different from than like his fellows, may be combined with either of two contrasting methods of investigation: the selective examination of many subjects (such as is done in testing many subjects to arrive at factors) versus the intense examination of a few subjects (exemplified in its extreme form by the single case study and in Ebbinghaus' classic investigation of verbal learning in himself as subject). As Marceil points out, theory and method can be combined in any of four combinations of these two positions on theory and methodologies.

The present research began with intensive study of many individuals (200) with the expectation of finding syndromes of specific variables which could be related to outcome. This expectation is based on a theory of similarity among subjects (i.e., that similar syndromes would lead to similar outcomes across subjects) but no such "similar syndromes" could be substantiated and, on the other hand, much of the richness of the intensive study of the *individual*, was lost in the use of the nomothetic method of analysis.

Nevertheless, some specific findings from the research did emerge from the analysis by group statistics and some of them have importance for clinical practice. They are discussed in this chapter along with those characteristics of the research design and certain clinical and life events that may have significantly affected the results.

In the two chapters to follow, we resort to the familiarity of our clinical orientation: in Chapter 6 we look behind the data scene at some of the children who did not adhere to the mainstream of the findings, such as those whose outcome was much better or much worse than would be predicted from their diagnoses. In Chapter 7 we elaborate on and interpret the therapy outcome results. These interpretive chapters are accompanied by case illustrations.

The last chapter of the book discusses the implications of the study for the place of child guidance, or, rather, of the outpatient clinical facility, in the delivery of mental health services to children and suggests a few changes in traditional policies and procedures within these services.

DISCUSSION OF FINDINGS

Although the findings from the data analysis confirm, in general, those of other recent, similar studies, their sparsity and the high incidence of improvement in the subjects at follow-up prompt these questions:

1. Were the subjects of this study really "children at risk?"
2. What childhood variables show continuity into adulthood or relate to adult adjustment? What characteristics differentiate those children who turn out well in adult social adjustment from those who do not?
3. What other factors, not immediately apparent in the statistical analyses, may have been influential in the more unexpected results of the study?

Were the Subjects Truly "At Risk"?

A little over half (54%) of the children in this study were rated, in adulthood, to be socially well-adjusted or only mildly maladjusted. Although this is a smaller proportion than has been found in most other research (usually about two-thirds are so designated), the fact that so many were not more seriously maladjusted at follow-up raises the possibility that the sample, as a whole, may not have been a high risk one to start with. Or, it might be that the clinic-referred children were no more disturbed, as a group, than a normative sample of their peers.

The literature supports both sides of this possibility: some surveys found little difference between referred and nonreferred children in schools

(Lapouse and Monk, 1958; Macfarlane et al., 1954; Shepherd et al., 1966); whereas others found that clinic children *were* deviant when compared to their classmates (Bower, 1960; Cowen et al., 1973; Glidewell et al., 1957).

The difference in results of the various surveys can sometimes be attributed to varying definitions of adjustment at outcome or the inclusion of varying degrees of disturbance. For example, the Shepherd et al. study (1966) *excluded* severely disturbed children from their clinic group which they then compared to a normal (i.e., nonreferred) school group matched for age, sex, and similarity of type of behavior. Within these limitations, their clinic children showed only a nonsignificant trend toward more severe ratings of behavioral disturbance initially and there were no significant differences in improvement rates between clinic-treated children and their nonclinic controls at follow-up some two years later.

By contrast, the Cowen et al. (1973) study identified children in the first grade and each year thereafter who "gave evidence of manifest or incipient maladaptation ranging from *"moderate"* to *"severe"* (italics ours) and these "red-tag" children (a third of the total school sample) functioned less effectively throughout the whole elementary school period than the "nonred-tag" children. More importantly, the red-tag group made up 68% of the 50 elementary school children listed over the ensuing 11-13 years in the County's Psychiatric Register. This high rate of psychiatric referral is doubly impressive because the 50 children who showed up in the Register were only 19% of the early identified (red-tag) children.

The Cowen et al. study is typical of mounting research evidence that 1) much of the behavior considered serious in childhood may not continue into adult pathology but that 2) a sample of children identified early as moderately to seriously disturbed will contribute a higher proportion of those destined for later clinically defined maladjustment than will their peers who were not so identified.

The data from both childhood and adulthood support the high risk status of the sample used in the present research project.

1. As children, they were referred to child guidance with symptoms and behaviors of many kinds and of varying degrees of seriousness. Ratings of the children in diagnostic conferences held after a comprehensive and intensive study of each child classed only 10% of them as healthy or only mildly disturbed. Various surveys of disturbance among school children in general place only 20 to 35% in the moderate and serious maladjustment categories as compared to the 90% of this sample (Wickman, 1928; Glidewell et al., 1959; Ullman, 1952).

    Moreover, the various indices of childhood disturbance including those recorded at the time of clinic contact, such as parents' and teachers' reports and clinical assessments and those independently produced from the follow-up staff's review of raw data from clinic charts, present a highly interrelated matrix of indices of disturbance (Table 7). (Some 80% of the 55 correlations are significant at the .05 level of significance or better.)

2. In adulthood, although rated much improved as a group over their childhood status, the sample still demonstrated a much higher degree of pathology than is present in the general population at this age. For example, the Midtown Manhattan Study (Srole, 1962) reports 15% of 20-29-year-olds in the "general population" to be "impaired," that is, having symptoms or behaviors which interfere "somewhat," "seriously," or "to an incapacitating degree" in life functioning. These categories of maladjustment are roughly comparable to the ratings of "moderate," "severe," and "incapacitating" which covered 46% of young adults in the present follow-up.

Psychiatric hospitalization figures on the follow-up are extremely high compared to the Manhattan Study, with 11% of the subjects having been hospitalized since clinic contact compared to under 1% reported for the Manhattan sample at this age level. This latter figure of 1% is quite consistent with the NIMH figures of 1971 for the age group 18-24 years (NIMH, 1971a).

The frequency of law violations (of a nontraffic kind) is also high. Of the young adults in this research, 19% admitted having been arrested in the period since clinic contact.

Both these subsamples, law violators and psychiatric inpatients, could be distinguished as having been rated more disturbed in childhood (social adjustment and intensity of disturbance) than those not reporting later arrests or hospitalization.

Thus, it seems safe to conclude that, within the limitations of the capability of the various independent sources to make judgments about disturbance, these 200 children did represent a high risk group.

What Childhood Characteristics Differentiated Well-Adjusted and Maladjusted Adults?

Most studies, including this one, can list few "continuous variables" in personality development whether they are simple personality traits such as those assessed in normative and longitudinal studies or more problem-focused variables such as those likely to be used with high risk children. Repeated long-term assessment such as that carried out by California University's Institute of Human Development (Hunt and Eichorn, 1972; Peskin, 1972) and the New York University Group (Thomas et al., 1968; Thomas and Chess, 1976) could come up with only a few characteristics which were consistent over time. Clarke and Clarke (1976), in reviewing longitudinal studies involving repeated assessments, suggest that

...prediction of later from earlier characteristics is on the whole poor, not primarily because of imperfect measurement, but because it is confounded both by discontinuities as well as by individual continuities which show variability over time (p. 21).

When the task was to determine which childhood variables were related to degree and kind of mental illness in adulthood, the results have been equally disappointing. In the Mellsop study (1972) where it was possible to follow up quite effectively children who were clinic patients and who became patients of the Victorian Mental Health Department in adulthood, the problem of prediction from childhood records was not resolved to the researchers' satisfaction. They concluded that they had found "little of predictive value" even though, as others have found, their clinic children turned out to be high risk in that they were greatly overrepresented among the adult population (4 times the expected number).

The present study has little additional data to bring to the issue of continuity. In only one area, that of life functioning in a social context, were specific behaviors, such as family relationships, assessed both in childhood and adulthood for the total sample. Of the five life functioning areas assessed, four showed significant but modest correlations ranging from .12 to .23. In a subsample of mother-subject pairs who complied with the follow-up interviewer's requests to check and return symptom lists about the subjects, there was further evidence for continuity of pathology in that the number and intensity of symptoms checked by mothers in childhood and adulthood correlated significantly. But these returns may not be representative of the total sample, since they included responses from only 34.5% of the subjects.

The issue of predictability was addressed through analyzing the relationships between many specific childhood variables and that of social adjustment in young adulthood. Out of 41 quantifiable childhood variables used in the regression analysis, only 14 (34%) were significantly related to outcome (at the .05 or better level). These 14 included a few items from the application data, such as social class and father's educational attainment, two items from the developmental data, several symptoms, several school behavior items, and the total number of such items checked, the diagnostic conference rating of intensity, the child's IQ, and, most significantly related of all, the childhood social adjustment rating.

Analysis of the "discrete" variables found several of them also to be related to outcome and there seems to be some logic and some precedent in other reported research for the meaning of these variables in prediction. They included a few variables which seem to denote a poor start in life such as low birth weight, boys who were not full-term at birth, and the young age at which the child's problems were first noticed.

Some other "predictors" were the kinds of antisocial behavior observed by teachers, especially, which find support in several studies relating antisocial behavior to poor prognosis. The relationship in the present follow-up between adult maladjustment and school behavior like poor peer relationships and temper displays is doubly important because this sample did not display, initially, the extremes of behavior seen in the Robins (1966) and Morris et al. (1956) samples of childhood. For example, one of the more important symptoms in terms of outcome in the Robins' study, serious truancy, was reported for only 7 of the children in this follow-up.

Alan is fairly representative of a small group of children in this study whose problems began with serious behavior such as truancy, petty thievery, lying, resistance to school authority, and association with a group of boys who were frequently in trouble at school and in the neighborhood. Alan had been expelled from a parochial school in the 7th grade and referred to the Clinic by his 8th grade teacher in a public school after a continuation of these same problems. Like mothers of many delinquent boys, Alan's mother was overly permissive and materially indulgent, tending to overlook and excuse his behavior. Father, who was much older than Alan's mother and lived mainly within a shell in order to avoid troublesome situations, punished Alan severely on those occasions when he was forced to intervene. The other children in this family have never been in trouble at school or in the community.

By the time of the follow-up interview, when Alan was 24, he had become a "social misfit." He met the interviewer outside his parents' home from which he had been evicted for the third or fourth time. He had stolen their television, radios, and other articles to get money for drugs and had broken doors and windows in anger when they refused to let him in or to give him more money. Mother, who had given to Alan too freely in childhood, had been forced to go back to work after retirement to replace the furniture and repair the house.

Alan said he never speaks to his parents except to try to get money. He spends his days "just bumming around" with a gang of fellows, sleeping in his old dilapidated car or in his parents' yard. He had been convicted for burglary and possession of drugs and, at the time of the interview, he had another court case pending for theft at a local department store. Alan has had one steady girl friend who quit him because of his drug addiction and his refusal to give up his gang activities.

In the interview, Alan expressed some desire to kick his drug habit (which he said he had picked up while in the Army overseas). But he also said he knew he wouldn't subject himself to the treatment necessary and that he didn't see how he could ever stay on a job should he ever begin work again. His pessimism over changing his life is reminiscent of his reaction to his therapy at the Clinic. After a few months in treatment, Alan just "decided I wouldn't go anymore and so I just didn't show up. They couldn't change my attitude." Mother had been seen also at the Clinic but father was unable to tolerate the therapeutic process.

Factors That May Have Affected the Number and Clarity of Findings

The findings of this research, some expected and others quite unexpected, may be better understood by taking into consideration 1) the characteristics of this particular sample in childhood and in adulthood, 2) the assessors and their instruments of assessment, and 3) the influence of life events, including therapy, intervening between childhood evaluation and follow-up interviews.

Sample-Related Variables

Age at Original Assessment. The success of prediction from childhood data seems to be highly dependent on the age of the children at the time the original data are collected. This finding has emerged repeatedly in longitudinal studies and in some follow-up studies. The weight of evidence now suggests that childhood is truly a time of flux in personality development when various kinds of behaviors and attitudes are being tried out in an attempt to cope with a variety of stresses presented by successive stages in development. *Only when* assessment occurs repeatedly along the way can the extent of this adaptive changing within children be appreciated.

Some of the other studies that find little relationship between childhood characteristics and adult outcome may do so because of the *age* of their childhood sample, whereas others do find relationships, such as the Robins group who chose, because of the availability of clinic records, to study a sample in which the median age was 13 years, an age which seems, from the results of longitudinal projects, to be the most "predictive" age for that particular kind of childhood disturbance (i.e., antisocial behavior). Livson and Peskin (1967) found the 11-13 age period most predictive in their follow-up and present rather convincing evidence for the changing nature, and even reversibility, of traits between successive ages such as preadolescence to adolescence.

In the present study, disturbances diagnosed at two age levels were related most clearly to poor adjustment in adulthood: the 4 to 6 year period and 12 years. (These ages emerged as important even without narrowing the *kinds* of problems.)

David's history demonstrates the importance of referral at a very young age or, more specifically, the fact that his disturbance was so severe that even at age 6 he was identified as being in need of clinic services. When referred by the school in his first grade for aggressive outbursts, continual fighting, and other unmanageable behavior, David had already been a problem for several years. Mother had placed him in a nursery school at age 3 because she couldn't cope with him at home. The nursery school teachers soon complained that David was impulsive, immature, and unable to get along with the other children. At home, he had set several fires before he was 4 years old.

David's parents were both emotionally impoverished people who came from upset families and seemed to lack resources of their own to meet David's needs. The Clinic recommended placement in a residential therapeutic center but the parents placed him, instead, in a children's institution which offered only an environmental treatment program. At age 11 he was returned to his parents. At 14 he made a serious attempt to kill his father and had to be hospitalized. At 18, after walking out of a posthospital foster placement setting, he returned home where he carries on his aggressive, impulsive behavior and keeps his parents in constant fear for their lives.

David's sociopathic behavior was entrenched by age 3. It was of such proportions and intensity that his young age did not allow the first grade teacher to dismiss his behavior as something which he would outgrow or which would pass away with time.

Age at Follow-up. Data from the follow-up interviews raise the possibility that some of the subjects were still too young for "permanent" adjustment patterns to have been established. A few researchers (Pollack et al., 1968; Peskin, 1972) have contacted subjects in late adolescence, young adulthood, and later adulthood and have reported major changes in adjustment still occurring between these points in time.

Haan (1972), reporting on a follow-up of normal subjects through comparison of their typologies in junior high school, in senior high school, as young adults, and in middle age, concludes that "not only are people very different from each other, but they move from adolescence to adulthood in very different ways" (p. 406). Only a few of the 5 male and 6 female "types" derived by Q-sort of personality characteristics displayed any consistency over the age spans studied, and the two showing the most continuity were types that were "persistently well adjusted psychologically." Moreover, no pathognomonic traits could be found to characterize the adolescents who later became disturbed. The *senior* high school years were especially nonpredictive to later adjustment.

Masterson (1967b) and the Morris group (1956), in separate studies of *disturbed* adolescents, report that when pathology is moderate to severe by middle to late adolescence, it persists into adulthood. Masterson, using "functional impairment" as his measure, found 62% of his 72 disturbed adolescent patients were moderately to severely disturbed five years later even with treatment. Morris et al., reevaluating as many as possible of their original group of 90 children who had been admitted as inpatients for aggressive behavior, found much consistency in pathology at ages 18, 25, and 30. They conclude, in fact, that if the adolescent had not adjusted well by age 18 he was not likely to do so (in the next 12 years). These two studies considered together support the premise that there seems to be continuity in good adjustment covering, in these studies, young adolescence into adulthood, and also in very poor adjustment when it is of an antisocial and/or psychotic nature. (Masterson found that his neurotics, even including character neurotics, were doing well in adulthood while those with schizophrenia and personality disorder were not.)

Many of the subjects (80) in the present study were still in high school or college when interviewed and only 55 had married. Some 106, or 53%, were still living with their parents. It is conceivable that for some of these young people, still in school and living at home, the experiences of separating from parents, supporting themselves financially, marrying, and raising a family might provide more stress and lead to further problems while, for others, such experiences might be beneficial.

While there were no significant differences in *overall* social adjustment between the different age groups at follow-up, the unexpected finding that the oldest age group, 23-28 years, had the highest percentage (22%) who were neither employed nor in school suggests that the follow-up results may have been different had the sample included more older subjects. Ideally, of course, follow-up projects would include repeated assessments from adolescence through adulthood in order to determine whether or not there *is* an age at which the individual personality becomes relatively stabilized.

Influence of the Sex Variable. The variable of sex has also been, until recently, neglected as a consideration in outcome research. Often only one sex has been studied (Roff, 1974; Bower and Shellhammer, 1960) and, more frequently, data from boy-girl samples have not been analyzed separately as to sex (Gersten et al., 1976; Thomas et al., 1968; Thomas and Chess, 1976; Pollack et al., 1966; Cowen, 1973). When, as in the Livson-Peskin (1967), Robins (1966), Mellsop (1972), Watt (1972), and Watt et al. (1970) projects, sex-related data are reported, quite different characteristics appear to be important for each sex.

In the Livson-Peskin research, for example, different sets of young adolescent variables were related to adult health in boys and girls. Boys who were extraverted and expressive but not irritable and girls who were independent and confident were found, in their 30s, to be relatively healthy. In the Mellsop follow-up (1972), males diagnosed personality and conduct disorders as children were overrepresented in the adult patient group while females so diagnosed were *under*represented. Watt's follow-up of schizophrenic adults found irritability, aggressivity, and defiance discriminated boys destined to become schizophrenic from their controls, whereas inhibited personality characterized the preschizophrenic girls. Gail Gardner (1967), on the other hand, found no relationship between aggressive childhood behavior and schizophrenic outcome for *either* sex. Instead, in males, neurotic symptoms in childhood had been recorded for adult male schizophrenics but not for females.

In the present research a few differences between males and females were noted in both childhood and adulthood. In addition, some childhood variables were related to adult adjustment for one sex but not the other, and other childhood variables had opposite effects in adulthood. For instance, more boys than girls came to the clinic; boys were more often referred by schools than girls. In childhood girls tended to show neurotic type symptoms, such as compulsivity, unusual fears, physical complaints, withdrawn behavior, and eating difficulties whereas boys manifested learning difficulties and restlessness. In adulthood, acting out behavior such as law violations and use of drugs and alcohol were far more prevalent in men than women. The childhood variables that showed differences between boys and girls were generally not related to adult outcome.

In considering the relationship between childhood characteristics and adult outcome, we found several variables were significant for boys, but not for girls and vice versa. Poor adult adjustment for boys was associated with external anxiety, selfishness, fighting, failure to get along with other children, preference for younger children, and accident proneness. In addition, boys' religion was related to adult adjustment with Catholic boys having poor outcome. Finally, several childhood variables were associated with poor adjustment for boys and good adjustment for girls. These included: disturbance in identity, low birth weight, prematurity, behavior problems, and having a Catholic mother.

These data are congruent with other research and highlight several factors. Those variables that show sex differences in childhood may not be important as predictors of adult outcome. Secondly, some variables that are associated with adult outcome are significant for both boys and girls, whereas others are important predictors for one sex and not the other. And finally, the significance of some childhood variables for predicting adult adjustment may be lost in a mixed sample when they have opposite effects in males and females.

Social Class and Family Intactness. Although these 200 children were tagged, by numerous indices, to be "at risk," they came from families which were, in general, adequate in several characteristics usually thought to be important to children's psychological well-being. Of the 200 children, 75% were being raised by both natural parents, 96% of the fathers and only 14% of the mothers worked full time, over two thirds of the fathers had at least a high school education, and 21% had bachelors' and advanced degrees. Most of the families owned their own homes and a majority of the fathers held white-collar or professional jobs.

These characteristics are quite different from those of the families of several other follow-up studies in which the clinic populations studied were largely from lower class, poorly educated families with a high incidence of broken homes. Thus, in the Robins' sample, only one third of the children were living with both natural parents at clinic contact and one third had spent at least six months in an institution or foster home. Of the fathers, 15% were unemployed and the employment status of another 10% was "unknown." One third were receiving financial assistance from social agencies and only 31% of the fathers had white collar and professional jobs or owned small businesses.

Although the families in this present study were at least average in social class and superficial stability, the parents were judged, on the basis of the information they gave at clinic contact, to have serious problems, individually and in their marital relationships. Only about 10% of the parents were rated as mature and/or emotionally stable and an even smaller number were said to have adequate capacity to cope with stress. Only 5% of the couples were described as having a good marital relationship. These negative evaluations may, of course, have been a function of assessor bias, a bias which is not uncommon when the assessor knows that the parents have a child referred for clinical service.

Since more than half the children were eventually rated as mildly or less maladjusted in adulthood, the intactness of their families may have operated in their favor and/or the parents' pathology may have been rated too harshly. (Ratings of the parents' pathology were not related significantly to ratings of maladjustment in their children at follow-up.)

Influence of Source of Referral. Recently there has been a growing recognition of the importance of the fact that children are usually brought or sent to clinics by agents other than themselves and that their problems are often not problems in their own eyes but only in those of the referring agents. This "societal" judgment of pathology may affect results of outcome research in at least two ways. First, the initial assessment of disturbance may be distorted by the concern of parents and/or other referral sources so that, for example, children may be considered to be more disturbed than they actually are. Secondly, the child's response to therapy may be adversely affected when he is not the one who is anxious about or suffering from his symptoms or behavior.

Some evidence relating to the first issue is available in this study in that the two sources of referral information, the parents' and teachers' reports of the child's behavior, often differed. It was evident from the data that the parents and teachers were each reporting the kinds of behaviors that bothered them and that their separate perceptions of a particular child were not always in agreement; in fact, the correlations between the total number of school items checked with both the total number of symptoms and with the sum of weighted symptoms checked by parents were two of the lower correlations in the interrater matrix.

Relationship of Diagnosis to Adult Adjustment. The findings of this study agree, in general, with those of several other studies that clinical diagnosis in childhood is an important predictor for adult social adjustment. The weight of evidence from the research literature now suggests that neurosis in childhood does not predict pathology or serious maladjustment in adulthood (Lewis, 1965; Robins, 1966; Kohlberg et al., 1972), while that of psychosis portends serious adult pathology although not, usually, of the same nature as the childhood "psychosis" (Robins, 1972).

The diagnosis of character disorder, especially of an antisocial kind, shows more continuity of behavioral correlates into adulthood than do the other diagnoses. Such is the case in the Morris et al. (1956) study of very aggressive inpatient children and in the Robins (1966) outpatient group where three fourths of the children were referred for serious antisocial behavior and nearly half were actually court referrals.

The present research sample encompassed a wide variety of diagnostic categories comparable to the types of children usually served in child guidance clinics at that time, except for the mentally retarded who were purposefully omitted. As was true of most similar clinics in the 1960s, neurosis was the most frequent diagnosis (50% of the sample), followed by personality (character) disorders, neurotic behavior disorders, borderline psychosis, and psychosis. Of these, ratings of adult outcome proved to be best for the two types of neurotic children and worst for borderline psychosis with character disorders midway between the neurotic and borderline adjustment. The diagnosis of "psychosis" as differentiated from borderline psychosis was applied to only 4 of the 200 children in the sample. Two of these 4 children made remarkable adjustments and brought the average adult rating of the four to a very low (good) level which, because of the few children involved, may be a spurious finding. (These two much improved children are discussed in Chapter 6.)

Childhood diagnosis was considered to be central to the main thesis of this research, that is, the prediction of adult adjustment from childhood variables. This diagnostic variable and the intensity of disturbance and adjustment ratings (both global and additive) were the only means of representing, in any unitary fashion, the "whole" person. For this reason, the findings on diagnosis are discussed in a separate chapter (6) in terms of a closer look at some children whose outcomes did or did not conform to what their childhood diagnosis would predict.

Two children are described here, in contrast one with another, to show the overall advantage of differential clinical diagnosis over presenting symptoms in predicting long-term social adjustment.

Alice and Marilyn were both referred to the Clinic because of a change in acadmic performance from very good to poor, school absenteeism, and general unhappiness.

In Alice's case, the presence of acute anxiety manifested in school phobia and the appearance of compulsive defenses led to a diagnosis of neurotic reaction. Treatment was offered but was refused by the family.

In Marilyn's case, loss of interest in school was accompanied by a corresponding loss of interest in friends and social activities, weeping, and loss of weight. She was also diagnosed as neurotic at the clinical conference and therapy was recommended but by the time it actually became available six months later, she had become disoriented, agitated, and even self-mutilating. A clinical reevaluation resulted in a change in diagnosis to that of borderline psychosis and she was hospitalized shortly thereafter. Since her initial hospitalization of two and one half years, she has had two subsequent hospitalizations, one recently.

At follow-up both girls were in their early twenties. Alice was finishing her last year of college, had a part-time job, a steady boyfriend, and many other friends including several close ones. Marilyn was married and had one child but was confined to her house in a rural area, had no friends, and lived in fear of her husband's brutality. She had left him twice but could not make it on her own and was no longer in touch with her parents. Although she was making a marginal adjustment outside the hospital, the interviewer found her to be far more disturbed than when she had first come to the Clinic at age 14.

Although these two girls had similar presenting problems, their personality structures were quite different. Alice's anxiety and inability to go to school was diagnosed correctly in childhood as a neurotic reaction, phobic in nature, but she had no thought disturbance nor other structural deviance. Once she had resolved the oedipal problems leading to her fears, personality development could proceed. Marilyn's fear of school, on the other hand, was occasioned by a misperception of the environment and illogical thought processes which affected her school performance and all her relationships. Even with therapeutic intervention, these ego deficits were not overcome.

This review of the importance of age, sex, social class, and diagnostic variables supports the opinion that the inclusion in the sample of children of both sexes, of all ages from 5 through 15, and of a wide variety of diagnostic categories may have resulted in the "canceling" out of outcome results specific to and mutually contradictory among age levels, the two sexes, and the various diagnoses.

For example, the inclusion of 100 neurotic children undoubtedly improved the outcome of the group as a whole. The higher predictability of later maladjustment at the 12-year-old level was certainly offset by the inclusion of children at other ages from which such prediction is less certain. The variety of the children in the study, on the one hand, and, on the other, the constriction of the sample in terms of the low incidence of severe pathology may have clouded the picture of outcome. Nevertheless, this variety was representative of the Clinic's population and is still typical of many community outpatient children's services. The research findings have practical implications for these services.

Assessor-Related Variables

Evaluations in Childhood. In addition to the influence of the specific nature of the sample used, the tracing of continuity of personality variables or of predicting pathology hinges, of course, on the reliability of the assessments. Although the different assessments of the children at the time of their referral to the Clinic were significantly intercorrelated and their evaluations in adulthood point to a high incidence of maladjustment compared to the general population, there was, nevertheless, disagreement among assessments which included parents,' school personnel's, individual clinician's, and conference judgments.

Parents and Teachers. As pointed out, parents as contrasted with teachers, were much harder on their children in that they reported more problems than did teachers, a finding which agrees with other studies such as Glidewell et al. (1959). In the present study, the number of problem behaviors teachers reported that they observed in children was significantly related to outcome while the number of such behaviors contained in parents' reports was not significantly related to outcome.

In the Cowen et al. research (1973), school personnel, consisting of both teachers and school mental health consultants, were able to "tag" a group of children as early as grades 1 to 3 moderately to seriously maladjusted and this group contributed a far greater percentage of clinical referrals to local psychiatric facilities in adolescence and young adulthood than did the other two thirds of the children not tagged as maladjusted. In Cowen's research, the children's peers were even more efficient in detecting those destined for later psychiatric service than were their teachers.

For some children the reports from the parents and from the school differed markedly as to the extent and severity of problems the child was displaying because of differences in perceptions of teachers and parents. In other instances these discrepancies were obviously based on an actual difference in the child's behavior at home and at school as, for example, when a studious, academically successful child used the home situation to get rid of aggression and frustration.

In Ronnie's case, however, it seems, now, that mother simply saw him in a very negative light, mainly because he reminded her of the husband who had mistreated and then deserted her. During the clinic evaluation, mother had checked nearly two thirds of the symptoms and behaviors on the clinic form, a number much above the average checked by the 200 mothers constituting the research sample. She described Ronnie as an angry, hostile boy whose demands on her were unreasonable and whose constant bullying of his brother kept the house in an uproar. In mother's eyes, he was sullen, trusted no one, had no friends, and was totally irresponsible.

Ronnie's school report, on the other hand, was only mildly negative. Although several teachers commented on his poor motivation, lack of confidence, and distractability, they described his behavior as generally satisfactory and a few of them commented on his "happy disposition," his "good sense of humor," and his "outgoing personality."

The research social worker, taking into account mother's negative report and the more positive school report and noting the special meaning that this boy had for his very disturbed mother, rated Ronnie as "moderately maladjusted." The psychologist and psychiatrist each rating independently from the social worker and from each other, also rated his disturbance as moderate.

At follow-up, Ronnie was doing very well and the interviewer, with no knowledge of these childhood ratings, rated Ronnie's adjustment as healthy. He was a 25-year-old college graduate and had an excellent position with much responsibility. After several traumatic moves back and forth between his divorced parents, Ronnie had moved away from both of them. Now he was living in a most attractive apartment, and had close friends and a steady girlfriend. The lack of motivation he had exhibited in childhood was nowhere to be found. "I'm not in Utopia, but I have no insurmountable problems." Even mother talked of Ronnie as a well-satisfied, happy young man.

Clinical Assessment. This project was designed to include uniform data from comprehensive clinical evaluation of children, data which have been rarely available in previous follow-up studies. It was thought that since this kind of intensive evaluation was regularly used at the Clinic as the basis for diagnosis and recommendations, it should also be an important source of the predictions from childhood to adult outcome. Kohlberg et al. (1972) saw the need for research including such an evaluation, especially to address the unanswered question of the importance of childhood emotional status and dynamics in the prognosis of adult mental health or illness. They conclude "From a practical point of view.... what is most urgently needed is a longitudinal evaluation of the current standard methods and concepts of psychodiagnosis, involving the psychiatric interview, the family interview and the projective tests" (p. 1272).

It was difficult to translate the clinic data available in psychological test productions, both psychometric and projective, and transcripts from psychiatric interviews into ratings based on psychodiagnostic concepts derived from dynamic theory. Variables were selected and defined which would correspond most closely to those usually addressed in the psychological and psychiatric reports of the regular clinic diagnostic evaluations. They included personality traits, measures of efficiency of ego functioning, and structural and dynamic concepts central to psychoanalytic theory.

These ratings from test and interview material covered 12 variables, a diagnostic label, and a rating of severity of disturbance. They were done independently by an experienced psychologist and psychiatrist for each child and without knowledge of any follow-up material about him. When the ratings were related to those of the life functioning of the subjects at follow-up, the results did not, in general, add much to those available from comparing life functioning in childhood derived from parent and school reports about the child with social adjustment in adulthood as rated by the follow-up interviewer. To summarize these finds from clinical assessment:

1. *The psychologists'* rating of severity of disturbance from testing did not relate significantly to ratings of adult functioning. Correlation between *psychiatric* ratings and adult adjustment almost reached the .05 level of significance but the correlation is so low that it has little practical significance.

2. The ratings of severity of disturbance and the diagnoses arrived at conjointly by professionals at a diagnostic conference were, on the other hand, one of the better predictors to adult adjustment. Although neither the psychologist's nor psychiatrist's material was productive separately toward meaningful prediction, the live collaboration at a conference at the time of clinic contact seems to result in diagnoses and estimates of degree of disturbance which have meaning for later adjustment. This is especially true for children judged, on the basis of social adjustment, to be severely maladjusted both at the time of clinic contact and in adulthood. Of these, 91% had been rated as clinically

disturbed at the conference. By contrast, only 49% of those children rated as least socially maladjusted at both points in time had been rated as seriously disturbed in their childhood by the conference team.

The diagnoses of the persistently most disturbed individuals were predominantly borderline, character disorders, and brain syndromes (totaling 55% of the most disturbed group) while the majority of the persistently *least* disturbed individuals (77% of the group) had childhood diagnoses of neurosis and transient or developmental difficulties.

3. Few of the individual items of childhood clinical assessment seemed to have importance for adult adjustment and those that did were usually sex-related and/or showed nonlinear relationship. For example, psychiatrists' rating of high *internal* anxiety was related to good adult adjustment and *external* (environmentally induced) anxiety to poor adjustment in adulthood, but only for males. The psychologists' rating of severity of disturbance was significantly related to adult adjustment for females only. It is difficult to organize the sparse and isolated findings from psychological and psychiatric assessment in any meaningful way.

4. One type of clinical assessment from childhood material, ratings of social adjustment, does relate significantly to adult adjustment (at the .001 level). While the higher degree of relationship between these assessments may be, in part, attributed to the similarity of the material used for the ratings, that is, in both cases life functioning of the individual, the two assessments were done by different raters and with complete independence of each other.

5. Clinical assessments on the same children also varied. Clinical psychologists rated the children mainly in the three middle categories on a 5-point scale (99% were in "mild," "moderate," and "severe"). Psychiatrists, too, avoided the extreme categories (healthy and incapacitated) but rated many more in the "mild" category (30%). The conference decisions agreed with psychologists in placing about one tenth of the children in the mild category but classified just under one third in the most extreme category, "incapacitated" and 28 and 31%, respectively, in the "moderate" and "severe" categories. Thus the conference diagnosis was more heavily weighted toward "severe" and "incapacitated" (62% in all) and it was only the conference diagnosis which was found to relate significantly to adult outcome.

While the correlation between intensity (of disturbance) and outcome was too low to be predictive, it does suggest that clinicians arrive at "better" judgments together than each would separately. Ratings of social adjustment had improved so much at follow-up, however, that it is necessary to search for plausible explanations.

The combination of findings just reviewed points to one hypothesis for the improvement in ratings in adulthood over childhood. It may be that parents become overconcerned and overreact to their children's behavior, perhaps because of the discomfort and fear it occasions in the parents. Teachers are not so personally close to the children and not so fully responsible for them and may be more objective because they have many more children with whom to interact and among whom they make comparisons. Parents bring their children and their concerns to the clinic, and clinicians, who tend to see pathology more easily than assets, agree with parents, diagnose most of the children as having moderate to serious disorders, and prescribe treatment for most of them.

In *some* cases, as it turns out later, both the parents and the clinicians, or one or the other, were justified in their concern. In *more* cases, however, their negative assessment may have been a result of not paying enough attention to the stage-specific nature of the problem behavior and/or to the resources the child might have to cope with problems. The rather general finding in research that intelligence and good early parental relationships are related to outcome supports the importance of resources.

Evaluations in Adulthood. The original design of this research had called for repetition of the intensive diagnostic study of each subject at follow-up. Because of limitations in funding, however, follow-up evaluations were restricted to a personal interview of the subject and of his or her mother.

The content of the follow-up interviews formed the basis for a social adjustment rating in five areas of life functioning and an overall social adjustment rating, six ratings in all which were as similar in content to the social adjustment ratings made from childhood social data as possible. The ratings of childhood and adulthood were found to be significantly correlated. The follow-up interviews also provided much factual information, some of which were important indices of life functioning, such as the incidence of hospitalization and law violations, and these were related to several childhood indices of disturbance.

The follow-up interviews probably did not tap underlying pathology very well, however, and an attempt to rate such pathology and personality characteristics from the single interview was not successful. (A second research project is underway to assess personality variables and pathology in selected subsamples of the original subjects.) The follow-up assessment was further limited by using only two sources of information, subjects and their mothers.

These limitations restrict the study to that of the outcome in social adjustment of 200 children referred to child guidance and intensively evaluated at that time. It is likely that some of them were still disturbed intrapsychically (that is, anxious, depressed, worried) without revealing these problems in the interview. Of course, the reverse is also possible but not as likely: the social adjustment interview, because of its limited nature, could result in ratings that were *more* pathological than would have been obtained by assessment of the "whole" person.

Importance of Intervening Events

It may be that the difficulty in predicting from childhood characteristics to adult adjustment is due, at least in part, to the influence of certain life experiences intervening between the two points in time. As research evidence accumulates, however, to cast doubt on previously favored theories of the continuity of personality development and of the great importance to be attached to experience in the first three years of life, the issue of the effects of intervening events, particularly of trauma and stress, has also been opened to debate. It now seems probable that life experiences intervening between early childhood and adulthood may counteract *or* reinforce earlier positive and negative experience and thereby influence adult adjustment in complex ways.

Research on the extent to which trauma and stress have unfavorable consequences for future development illustrate the complexity of the issue. Studies on the effects of loss, separation, deprivation, and isolation suggest that while immediate negative effects are discernible, long-range effects are less certain. Moreover, as more research has been done, it becomes apparent that the multiple variables associated with a particular event influence its effects. For example, when a child loses a parent, his response to separation is influenced by the prior relationship to the parent as well as the type of parenting received after the separation. Rutter (1976) found that differential effects of separation were related to family circumstances. For example, psychological disturbance in children separated from their parents was associated with separation from parents who were in a conflictual marriage, whereas children separated from parents who had an adequate marriage did not show disturbance.

A somewhat similar view, based on clinical impressions, was presented by Goldfarb (1970) who suggested that children's deterioration following residential treatment was associated with disturbance in family interaction whereas improvement was related to favorable family situations. Thus, the effects of separation from the residential treatment center and incorporation into a family varied considerably.

It appears that particular events in a child's life influence development but the nature of that influence is related to prior experiences, the meaning of the event for the particular child, the supports available to the child at the time, and subsequent life experiences. Evidence for this viewpoint comes from two kinds of observations: the resiliency of the human organism and the aftermath of crisis intervention.

Kagan (1976) suggests that the infant is resilient and the effects of early experiences are reversible. In summarizing findings from a variety of research efforts, Kagan concludes:

> The data offer no firm support for the popular belief that certain events during the first year can produce irreversible consequences in either human or infrahuman infants. (p. 121)

The resilience of the human organism and its potential for growth are supported by observations derived from work in crisis intervention. In coping with crises, some individuals not only overcome the negative effects of stress but grow noticeably in the process. During exposure to stressful events, one experiences disequilibrium and responds by trying to regain homeostasis. These efforts may lead to reestablishment of precrisis functioning or may stimulate new growth as adaptive mechanisms are developed. One crucial factor in this process of crisis resolution is the availability of adequate supports in the environment. Thus, various negative life events or experiences may contribute to later maladjustment, may have only temporary effects, or may even be growth-producing.

In our follow-up study, the interviewers noted and were impressed by the number of young adults who reported that they made a decided turn toward better adjustment upon making certain changes in their lives such as leaving home and an overprotective mother, finding satisfaction in academic or occupational achievement, marrying or forming a relationship with a father- or mother-substitute such as a teacher or employer. Therapy has been elevated by clinicians to a position of eminence among "intervening events" which also may be expected to affect future adjustment.

Two case histories illustrate contrasting effects of intervening life events: Roger has successfully adapted and Dale has deteriorated over the years intervening between clinic referral and follow-up. Factors important in Roger's successful adjustment include separation from mother, therapy, and meaningful relationships with a male teacher, peers, and a girlfriend. In contrast, Dale was unable to cope with and master two deaths in the family and the loss of his first job after college. The absence of meaningful relationships seems to be a contributing factor in Dale's deterioration since it left him without a potential source of support.

When first seen, Roger was a very upset and behaviorally disorganized 10-year-old. His mother had brought him to the Clinic at the suggestion of the school social worker who said he was in continual difficulty. He was hitting other children, interrupting classroom activities, and paying little attention to the teacher. At home he was anxious and very depressed. He alternated from the depths of being nobody, inadequate and unloved, to being Superman who would try anything to show his prowess. His depression was so severe at times that he talked of suicide and made some moderately serious suicide attempts.

Although he had always been a bright, sensitive, and emotional child, Roger's anxiety seemed to snowball after his parents' divorce and his mother's subsequent "nervous breakdown." Roger, the oldest of five children, had been close to his father who served as a buffer against the intensity of an hysterical mother who had singled Roger out for a symbiotic folie-a-deux attachment. Roger tried and, of course, failed at filling the absent father's role and then felt extremely guilty and worthless.

Roger's sense of worthlessness mounted when mother married again. The stepfather was a new oedipal threat without providing any of the support or nurturance that his natural father did. It was at this time that clinic service was sought.

The clinic recognized Roger's severe neurotic disturbance and the real threat of suicide he was under. The staff was also so impressed by the severity of his mother's disturbance, however, that they recommended inpatient psychiatric treatment for Roger and warned, in the diagnostic conference, that "as long as the patient remains with mother. . . he has the potential to develop (as had mother) into a 'professional patient.' "

Roger was placed in a psychiatric inpatient unit for children and therapy was initiated with a male psychiatrist who saw him frequently for the year he was there and afterward on a once- or twice-a-week basis through age 15. This relationship meant a great deal to Roger and he made some progress. According to his recollection at follow-up, however, he remained depressed and intensely anxious until he came to a realization in therapy that he could never get well until he left the web of the seductive-hostile relationship with his mother. With help from an uncle he accomplished the separation.

The process of individuation which therapy had begun gradually gained momentum with the separation. Roger began to make use of his excellent intellectual assets in the academic area, he made friends, and he found new interests in music, art, and community activities. Another intervening event of importance seems to be the interest that one of his college professors took in him and the stimulus it provided for his professional career. (Interestingly, remnants of his own early depression are evident in his choice of a part-time job, while in college, as a counselor to terminally ill patients.)

Another salutory life experience has been his relationship and engagement to a stable, giving, and professionally effective young woman. As

Roger expressed it to the follow-up interviewer, "I have finally faced my problems; I know the misery of anxiety but I no longer fear it so much that I have to run from it into omnipotence or self-destruction."

In addition to the influence of life experiences, Roger's history also illustrates the unpredictability of outcome when the illness was largely in the parent at time of clinic referral. Roger was indeed seriously disturbed in childhood and his disturbance was even internalized. But his trauma was so linked to mother's illness and her need to draw this child into it, that even with therapy, he could not overcome the downhill pull as long as he remained with her.

The follow-up interview with mother shed further light on Roger's development and the importance of his separation from her. Mother's severe disturbance (schizophrenia) was evident in her bland affect, regressed appearance, childlike verbalization, and her account of years of therapy and periodic hospitalizations. In describing Roger's childhood, her emphasis on enjoyment in playing with the children conveyed a sense of being a child with her children and reflected her inability to see the children as individuals separate from herself.

Roger's history also illustrates the complexity of influences between clinic evaluation and follow-up and the difficulty of sorting out any *single* variable as most important.

Dale was referred to the clinic at age 13 because of parents' concern about his "nervousness." He had developed many obsessive-compulsive symptoms including handwashing rituals and excessive religiosity. The development of symptoms was related to two deaths, those of a younger sibling and a grandparent within a period of several weeks, accompanied by the addition of a remaining grandparent to the household. This grandparent was ill and required considerable care by Dale's mother. Thus, he experienced real losses and the added stress of mother's emotional withdrawal.

Dale was able to perform well academically in high school and college but had no friends. Although he participated in sports activities, he did not develop friends through these activities. Upon college graduation Dale acquired an appropriate job but, a year later, the company went out of business and for the past year Dale has been unemployed. He continues to live at home, an isolated schizoid personality. At follow-up Dale stated he does not have close friends and cannot trust people.

At the time of clinic contact Dale was considered to be in need of intensive psychotherapy to deal with an obsessive-compulsive neurosis. Three years of treatment were not effective in interrupting his symptoms and halting a regressive trend. Dale was seen individually for one year and he stated that it was "an impersonal deal." Next he had a year in group therapy. Here Dale felt he could "cover up" and "fake it" as he sat without saying much. A third year of treatment utilized family therapy. This was helpful to parents but not to Dale.

In Dale's case, the traumatic effects of the deaths of two family members stimulated a pattern of withdrawal, isolation, and lack of trust. Dale's capacity to relate remained impaired during three years of therapy and his distancing interfered with efforts to help him deal with the unacceptable feelings he experienced in relation to deaths. Dale now sees himself at age 25 as an "unhappy person," a "perpetual pessimist." He expects to be hurt and states his life is focused on survival. He expects the worst and if something good happens, he doesn't allow himself to become too happy because he's sure it won't last.

Thus, these two young men both experienced difficult life situations. One was able to use a variety of relationships to promote growth and maturity while the other was unable to use therapy or any other type of relationship to halt his pattern of withdrawal and isolation.

Follow-up Study of Intervening Life Events. Since the long-range influence of intervening events on adult adjustment varies and the same events seem to have different effects on different people, we decided to make an effort to obtain more information about such experiences. Consequently, additional interviews were conducted with a subsample of 40 subjects who participated in the original research. These subjects were interviewed one to two years after the first period of follow-up data collection.

The subsample was composed of 10 subjects whose social adjustment ratings were clustered around the mean in both childhood and adulthood, 15 subjects whose rank order social adjustment ratings in childhood and adulthood had shifted from most to least disturbed, and 15 subjects whose ratings had shifted from least to most disturbed. Subjects were asked to identify the *most* important events or experiences that had influenced their development, either positively or negatively; then to identify other events that had specifically positive influences and those that had specifically negative influences and to state the ages at which these events occurred.

The 40 subjects altogether identified 209 events and labeled each as positive or negative. A few experiences were labeled mixed in effect, that is, the subject considered the experience as having simultaneous positive and negative meaning, or that it was felt initially as negative but had long-term positive effects or vice versa. The frequencies with which various events were identified are contained in Table 20.

The experiences fall into three categories, those generally perceived as having a positive effect, those with a negative effect, and those which were both positive and negative. Those experiences most often viewed as positive seem particularly relevant to young adults and their developmental tasks, the achievement of independence and the completion of education, or the continuation of work toward educational goals. These were most often expressed in specifics such as "leaving home and being on my own," "learning to be independent," and "graduating from high school," or "going to college."

Table 20. Important Life Events

Event	Total	Positive	Negative	Mixed
Rel. w/friends	31	13	18	—
Rel. with parents	26	11	11	4
School	25	6	16	3
Employment	22	11	10	1
Self-esteem	19	8	9	2
Independence	13	12	1	—
Complete educ.	12	12	—	—
Group experience	12	8	2	2
Loss	12	1	10	1
Marriage	10	5	3	2
Counseling	7	5	2	—
Have child	5	3	1	1
Trauma	5	—	5	—
Specific living pl.	5	3	2	—
Other	5	3	2	—
Total	209	101	92	16

In addition, group experiences, usually occurring prior to age 16, were also viewed positively: belonging to scouts, an athletic team, or the school band.

Those experiences most frequently viewed negatively included loss of a parent through separation or death, breakup of love relationships, and a death of a close friend or relative. Traumatic events also perceived negatively were serious illness of a family member and physical attack (robbery, rape) on the subject.

School experiences were frequently identified as important and were often judged to be negative. Included in these negative school experiences were frequent change of schools, poor achievement, and negative attitudes of school personnel. Positive school experiences included relationships with teachers and enrollment in private schools.

Of particular importance in the statements about schools are the different attitudes toward the same type of experience. Three subjects viewed a change in schools positively, two viewed the event negatively, and two felt the initial effect of changing schools was negative but the long-term effect was positive. Obviously, the impact of this experience is determined not so much by the factor of change but whether or not the new situation was more or less satisfying than the previous one, that is, whether the change constituted a gain or a loss for the individual child.

Two types of experiences, relationships, or interaction with friends and with family members were most frequently identified as being important to the young adults. Slightly more of these experiences were perceived as negative than positive. Such things as parental or sibling support, guidance, and encouragement were regarded as having a beneficial effect. Negative family influences included strict discipline, father's alcoholism, and abuse.

The influence of peer relationships in the developmental process is evident in the high frequency with which this area is mentioned as important. Half of the 40 subjects specified relationships with friends as important influences in their life and this area was mentioned for all age periods. Subjects identified the experience of having friends, establishing new friendships, acquiring a best friend, or establishing a love relationship as positive. As expected, the absence of friends and rejection or ridicule by peers were experienced negatively.

The number of positive as compared to negative events considered important differed with age ($X^2 = 11.47$, 4df, $p < .05$). The highest proportion of positive experiences occurred between ages 15 and 18 and the highest proportion of negative ones between ages 6 to 11 and 19 to 21 (Table 21).

Table 21. Age at Which Important Life Events Occurred[a]

Age (in years)	Positive Event (N = 98)	%	Negative or Mixed Event (N = 104)	%
6-11	19	9.4	36	17.8
12-14	12	5.9	20	9.9
15-18	28	13.9	15	7.4
19-21	24	11.9	21	10.4
Over 21	15	7.4	12	5.9

[a]$X^2 = 11.47$, 4 df, $p < .05$.

The types of experiences considered to be important differed by age but not to a significant degree. Relationships with friends and experiences affecting self-esteem were important at all ages from 6 to 28 years. The frequency with which family relationships were considered important gradually decreased from fifteen in the 6 to 11 year age span to none in the over 21 years group. From 15 years on, educational accomplishment, independence, and employment are stressed, choices which seem appropriate for this age group.

It was expected that examination of intervening life events might contribute to our understanding of factors influencing adult adjustment. Certainly the 40 subjects interviewed reported experiences and events that are theoretically relevant to adult adjustment. However, the number and type of events, their evaluation as positive or negative, and the age at which they occurred did not differentiate the three groups in the subsample: subjects whose social adjustment ratings in childhood and adulthood had shifted from least to most disturbed, those whose ratings remained at the mean, and those whose ratings shifted from most to least disturbed.

This analysis of the findings on intervening life events suggests that although young adults can identify life events which they believe to be important influences in their lives, the exact nature of an event and the perception of it varies among individuals. Moreover, the same type of experience may contribute to growth and maturity in one person or to maladjustment in another, or may have no long-term effect in others.

CHAPTER 6

Diagnosis in Childhood as it Relates to Adult Adjustment

The application of diagnostic labels to disturbed children was a logical sequel to the belief that adult disorders have their beginnings in childhood and to the movement, within this century, to develop more comprehensive and detailed systems of classifying these disorders in adults. In their recent review, Silverman and Ross (1972) cite Cramer's (1959) observations that Kraepelin's original classification in 1904 contained no mention of children.

Since Kraepelin's time and throughout the ensuing worldwide efforts to arrive at an adult diagnostic system which psychiatrists everywhere can agree upon and use, children's disorders have been recognized, at most, through the addition of a few labels that pertain only to children. Most children's disorders were relegated to coverage by adult nomenclature much as children in poor families wear the hand-me-downs of older siblings. Thus, the first *Diagnostic and Statistical Manual of Mental Disorders* which appeared in 1952 referred only to "adjustment reactions of childhood and of adolescence" under the heading of "transient situational disorders." Even in the *DSM II* (American Psychiatric Association, 1968) which represents a concerted effort by American psychiatry to collaborate with the World Health Organization in developing a system to reflect the fact that "people of all nations live in one world," slight recognition is accorded the *little* people of the world. The only additional classifications dealing specifically with the disorders of childhood and adolescence were "special symptoms, behavior disorders and, mental retardation and schizophrenia, childhood type."

The problem with the earlier classification systems is not only that they neglect children and adolescents but, more importantly, that the classifications arise essentially out of a medical model of disease entities and are based mainly on descriptive and behavioral data. The retention of the medical model is criticized in a recent issue of the *American Psychologist* by Schacht and Nathan (1977) as part of their appraisal of the latest revision of the psychiatric *Diagnostic and Statistical Manual of Mental Disorders, DSM III* (APA, 1977).

Child psychiatry, from the earliest days, was largely dynamic child psychiatry and from the days of Freud onward it began to recognize the

importance of "structural, dynamic, economic, genetic and adaptive characteristics" in diagnosis. According to the analysts, symptoms and behaviors can
have different meanings and importance for prognosis according to underlying reasons for their being. But even more influential in the task of
classification was the psychoanalytical belief in the need to attend to
development: the *gradual* maturing of the organism's structures and functions
so that a description of a child at any point in time could only be meaningful in
terms of his current status on several developmental scales and their
interrelationships. Added to this belief was the recognition that environmental factors are important in the production and in the understanding of
pathology. These considerations have led to the formulation of multi-axial
systems of diagnosis such as those of Rutter (1972) and Anthony (1958).

Curiously, two divergent movements are occurring simultaneously among
those providing clinical services to children, one urging more and better
attention to diagnosis, and the other considering all attempts at classification
impossible and/or unjustifiable. The first position, espoused chiefly by child
psychoanalysts, calls for a more intensive effort at diagnostic formulation to
include "descriptive—clinical, genetic and dynamic dimensions" (GAP, 1966,
p. 176). This effort culminated in the *GAP* classification advanced in 1966
by the Committee on Child Psychiatry of the Group for the Advancement of
Psychiatry. Listed as "psychopathological disorders of childhood" are nine
categories and one for "healthy responses," each with lengthy definitions. The
classes of disorders include some of those in DSM II: psychoneurosis,
psychoses, personality disorders, psychophysiologic disorders, mental retardation, and brain syndromes, but subdivide these classes into disorders
peculiar to children and add healthy reponses, reactive disorders, and developmental deviations. Items from a separate "symptom list" may be added
to each diagnosis.

The *GAP* classification of children's disorders with their definitions
represents a vast improvement over the previous adult-oriented systems.
However, as the Committee on Child Psychiatry points out, it falls far short of
the eventual goal of a "synthesis of the clinical picture, the psychodynamic and
psychosocial factors, genetic considerations regarding the level of origin, the
major etiological forces, a concise prognosis and the appropriate method of
treatment" (GAP, p. 209). Indeed, it is unlikely that any such synthesis will
ever be possible in a classification system as such.

The GAP report claims only to have developed a "clinical-descriptive
system," i.e., operational definitions of clinical categories which do imply,
however, "some inferences regarding etiology, prognostic outlook and
treatability . . ." (GAP, p. 209). As an addendum to their report, the
Committee provided an outline for a more complete diagnostic formulation.
In addition to descriptive-clinical and dynamic-genetic factors, it includes

parent-child relationships, family interaction, demographic, and other socio-cultural influences.

This *GAP* report is, in essence, the same sort of formulation that has engaged the efforts of the Hampstead staff over the last few decades. While recognizing the importance of symptoms in diagnostic classification, these analysts have attempted to "bridge the gap" between the contrasting approaches of descriptive symptomatology and metapsychological formulation. It is the latter metapsychological approach which has furthered the analysts' therapeutic efforts and which, according to Anna Freud and her co-workers, must be pursued in research on the development of personality and pathology. Nevertheless, this group, too, recognizes that they are advocating an extensive diagnostic study of each individual which can hardly be summarized in a single diagnostic term. One section of their *Diagnostic Profile* (A. Freud, 1962) attempts to "reassemble the items (of the profile) and to consider them in a clinically meaningful assessment," that is, to decide upon a diagnosis. These diagnoses are cast in a developmental framework as follows:

1) that in spite of current manifest behavior disturbances, the personality growth of the child is essentially healthy and falls within the wide range of "variations ot normality";

2) that existent pathological formations (symptoms) are of a transitory nature and can be classed as by-products of developmental strain;

3) that there are permanent regressions which on the one hand, cause more permanent symptom formation and, on the other hand, have impoverishing effects on libido progressions and crippling effects on ego growth. According to the location of the fixation points and the amount of ego-superego damage, the character structure or symptoms produced will be of a neurotic, psychotic or delinquent nature;

4) that there are primary deficiencies of an organic nature or early deprivations which distort development and structuralization and produce retarded, defective, and non-typical personalities;

5) that there are destructive processes at work (of organic, toxic or psychic, known or unknown origin) which have effected, or are on the point of effecting, a disruption of mental growth. (A. Freud, 1977, p. 10).

Both the GAP and the Hampstead systems of classification have been influenced in a major way by development of a theory of ego psychology. The gradual formation of the ego with its progressive refinement of functions can be viewed as the focal point around which a classification system for children's disorders can be built.

Settlage (1964) writes that the major variables in a meaningful classification are directly or indirectly represented in the ego and its functions. He points out the importance, in children, of the timing of traumatic experiences in relatior to the stage of ego development, to determine, for example, whether the disorder will be a psychosis or neurosis. Settlage advocates that the major categories be redefined in terms of stage-specific conflicts with symptoms and defenses appropriate to the particular stages of ego and psychosexual development. This viewpoint is compatible with the diagnostic progression of Anna Freud given above.

Those who have adopted a nihilistic viewpoint toward diagnosis point to the lack of predictive validity of diagnostic conclusions, to their irrelevance in prescribing treatment, to the social dangers inherent in "labeling" people, especially children, and to the impossibility of casting into any diagnostic label individuals with a diversity of characteristics. Those who object to a dependence on diagnosis include such strange bedfellows as psychoanalysts and Rogerian and behavioristic psychologists and psychiatrists (see, for example, Arthur, 1969; Breger, 1968; Kanfer and Saslow, 1965, 1969). Moreover, child-analytic *therapists* have traditionally discounted the need for diagnosis before psychotherapy. Their recent concern for developing diagnostic categories stems from their *research* interest in personality development.

DIAGNOSTIC CLASSIFICATIONS USED IN THE FOLLOW-UP PROJECT

At the time this research project was launched, the Clinic had been providing for more than ten years a highly formalized diagnostic service for each child and his or her family, employing at least a social worker, psychologist, and psychiatrist in the workup. In 1960, in planning for this prospective follow-up study, the Clinic introduced a form to record in a consistent manner decisions arising from the diagnostic conferences held at the conclusion of each diagnostic study.

This form included primary and additional diagnoses, intensity and chronicity of disturbance, prognosis for improvement and major clinical recommendations, both "practical" and "ideal." Each conference chairman was provided the Diagnostic Guidelines (Appendix A) to aid him and the professional team in making a diagnosis.

The particular classification of disorders upon which the Diagnostic Guidelines were based was a revision and extension of the *DSM I* classification which, as pointed out, is applicable mainly to adults. The Clinic revised it chiefly by: adding the category "normal" and elevating the subcategory "transient situational personality disorders" to the separate category "transient or developmental problems" specifically related to age-specific adjustment problems; adding the category "neurotic behavior disorder" to take care of the fact that some behavior (character) disorders still include guilt and anxiety; adding the separate category "borderline psychosis"; and including infantile autism and symbiotic psychosis in the category "psychotic reaction" along with schizophrenic reaction, psychotic affective disorder, and other psychotic reactions; using a single category for brain syndrome (rather than acute and chronic); and providing a place to cite the cause as well as the degree of mental deficiency.

Neither the *GAP* nor the Hampstead *Diagnostic Profile* were available at the time these guidelines were initiated at the Clinic. As described in Chapter 3, the conference diagnosis itself was only a final step in a long process of diagnostic study by a professional team whose dynamic formulations included specific conclusions on a host of individual personality and family interaction variables. These formulations were based on the same genetic-dynamic approach that produced the GAP and Hampstead profiles.

In the research reported here, the diagnostic formulation and diagnosis used in the statistical analysis were provided by research psychiatrists and psychologists at follow-up (in the 1970s) but were based on the interview and test protocols in the Clinic's records from childhood. These later diagnoses were made according to *GAP* classification. The Clinic guidelines, unlike the *GAP* system, include a separate category for neurotic behavior disorder and borderline psychoses. The use of each of these diagnoses seems to have had meaning insofar as outcome is concerned.

RELATIONSHIP OF CHILDHOOD DIAGNOSIS TO OUTCOME

In spite of the imperfections of diagnostic classification, there is evidence from research that diagnoses in childhood have some meaning in terms of subsequent adjustment. Thus, while the results from a majority of follow-up studies of outpatient clinic children point to an improvement rate of about 60 to 70% with or without treatment, exceptions to this optimistic prognosis are reported from studies of a few particular diagnostic categories and of extreme disturbances. Such is the case in the Morris, Escoll, and Wexler study of very aggressive inpatient children (1956) and in Robins' (1966) outpatient group, most of whom had been in court for serious delinquency. Psychotic children, also, are likely to be seriously disturbed as adults (Bender, 1969; Lotter, 1974).

Much of the follow-up and follow-back research agrees as to the relationship of childhood diagnosis to adult outcome. Briefly, diagnoses of childhood psychosis and severe character disorders including sociopathy are associated with adult pathology. Few report neurosis as leading to serious adult maladjustment and in some studies neurotic children were not distinguishable at follow-up from "normal" controls (e.g., Mellsop, 1972).

One researcher (Waldron, 1976) found that for only 17, or 40%, of his former neurotic children was adult illness definitely diagnosable. These 17 adults with illnesses diagnosable by the *CAPPS* (Current and Past Psychopathology Scales) were composed of 9 neurotics, 6 personality disorders, and 2 psychotics. Waldron contrasted these with 20 controls matched for childhood variables who showed *no* diagnosable adult illness according to *CAPPS*. He says little in his report, however, about the 25 neurotic children (60%) who had no diagnosable illness as adults.

In the present research, also, clinical diagnosis in childhood was quite logically related to social adjustment in adulthood except for one category, psychosis, which included only four children and two of these improved dramatically. The outcomes for the other categories agree, in general, with the findings of several other studies. The degree of maladjustment in adulthood was related to childhood diagnoses of borderline psychosis, brain syndrome, character disorder, neurotic behavior disorder, neurotic reaction, and transient reactions in childhood in descending order.

The existence of rich clinical records from childhood affords an opportunity to look backward to search for possible bases for outcomes that did or did not conform to expectations for particular diagnostic categories.

Although the relationship between diagnoses and outcome was significant and agreed in general with other research, there were children in each diagnostic category who did not "turn out" as would be expected from their diagnosis. Several hypotheses can be offered for this. One, of course, is that they have been misdiagnosed in childhood. It is true that for some cases the conference diagnosis, which is the one used in the following case illustrations, did not agree with the psychiatric and/or psychological diagnoses assigned by the research clinicians. There were other cases of unexpected outcome, however, in which there was consensus among the three judgments regarding diagnosis, at least as to the major category.

The first group of children, those who may have been misdiagnosed, may provide information about the "accuracy" (in terms of better predictability) of one or another of the diagnoses in light of the outcomes; the clinical records and follow-up information about the second group of children should contain the seeds for hypotheses as to why they deviated from expectations. It could be, for example, that assets in the child or fortuitous circumstances in the environment were present but not given sufficient weighting in the diagnostic formulation or that disorders which seemed to be internalized can be recognized from the advantage of hindsight to have been only reactive or transitory.

The possible effects of psychotherapy are considered in this chapter where appropriate, but this issue is treated specifically in a separate chapter on treatment outcome.

The case illustrations which follow represent, in part, an attempt to use clinical records to make sense out of unexpected results. The diagnosis that resulted from team discussion at the clinical conference in childhood is the one selected for the case illustrations.

The Four "Psychotic" Children

The diagnosis of "psychosis" (as distinct from borderline psychosis) was not lightly conferred at the time of the clinic contact. Only four children, or 2%, of the 200 in the research sample were so designated, a number which cannot be considered excessive even for a clinic population. The number is, however, too small to allow for any generalizations as to characteristics in childhood which make for continuity of psychosis into adulthood. Instead, some insight as to the differences in outcome among these four children may be gained from a review of each of the four clinical syndromes. Possible reasons for good outcomes for two children and poor outcomes for the other two range from questionable diagnosis to positive early life experience.

Two of the four children are still quite disturbed as adults, one rated as moderately and one as seriously maladjusted. Both Tom and Wanda display some continuity in the pathology noted in their childhood.

Tom, who is a nervous, effeminate 18-year-old at follow-up, lives at home with his parents and has been under psychiatric care for the last three years. Although he is a senior in high school, his grades are much below average, he has no friends—"the kids make fun of me, I'm strange"—and he can't get along with his teachers—"they scare me." Tom calls himself "paranoid" and feels he will "explode" some day. He thinks his parents, his teachers, and his schoolmates are "unfair" but then he also thinks of himself as "worthless." He spends his time at home listening to music and his sole interest at school is in electronics—"my electronic equipment keeps me company." Tom told the interviewer he expects never to marry "because no one will want me."

When referred to the Clinic at 7 years of age, Tom was not doing his work at school and could not get along with the other children. His behavior was often autistic and bizarre. For example, his teacher said he was fascinated by flies and electric fans and followed their movements with his eyes and his hands.

In the Clinic examination, there was no mistaking his severe pathology. He told openly of his fears of total destruction, freely associated in a chain of "clang" phrases, fused one idea with another, and, in general, used language in an autistic, conflict-oriented manner. He tested in the Dull Normal range of intelligence and, because of his clumsiness, a slight speech impediment, and very poor concentration, he was referred for a neurological examination and an EEG. The results were "indeterminate but suspicious of mild organicity." When he was placed in the Clinic school for disturbed children, however, it became apparent that he was not inferior intellectually and that his motor and attention difficulties could easily be accounted for on an emotional basis.

There was good agreement among the Clinic's diagnosticians that this boy was psychotic at 7 years of age; they disagreed only as to whether he should be called borderline or truly schizophrenic and whether or not there was any organic basis for his pathology. He stayed at the Clinic school for one year during which he had weekly psychotherapy while his mother participated in group therapy. His subsequent history has been one of severe problems in every area of functioning accompanied by personal anxiety and loneliness. He was referred for psychiatric treatment in young adolescence because of panic attacks at school and was receiving medication on a psychiatric basis at follow-up.

Tom's pathology has changed little in the last 11 years before follow-up. He is and was a victim of "pananxiety," feels extremely depressed and worthless, and has almost no social relationships. His preoccupation with things electric has persisted as the one friendship he has. Mother thinks therapy has helped Tom to function, albeit on a marginal level, and she is probably right.

Wanda's record illustrates a problem that may also apply to children in diagnostic categories other than hers.

The diagnosis of schizophrenic reaction, chronic, undifferentiated type which resulted from the Clinic conference was a compromise one. The psychiatrist who interviewed her at 13 years of age thought she displayed more of a character disorder but might later have a psychotic breakdown, and the psychologist who tested her described an inadequate personality with few resources. The research psychologist and psychiatrist, too, using childhood clinic protocols, did not call her schizophrenic but both described her extreme dependency, the psychologist calling it a dependent personality disorder and the psychiatrist calling it neurotic in nature.

Wanda represents an example of difficulty encountered when personality is in a stage of upheaval because of recent trauma and when it is difficult to determine the degree of possible permanent ego impairment. *All* the diagnosticians were seeing the same inadequate, overly dependent 13 year-old girl who was quite illogical when she talked about her mother who had died two years earlier. Mother had been psychotic and had been hospitalized repeatedly from the time Wanda was an infant. Moreover, Wanda was sleeping with her mother at the time of her death. After this trauma, Wanda became extremely depressed, talked bizarrely about mother as if she were still alive, and began to fail in school work.

The question at the diagnostic conference was, How much regression had already occurred? A diagnosis of "schizophrenic reaction" seemed to be suited to this uncertainty over the degree of disorganization. Supportive therapy was recommended but only three sessions, one each month, were held before the stepmother withdrew Wanda from clinic service.

During the follow-up interview when she was 23, Wanda said she had seen a private psychiatrist for a period of six months when she was 14 but didn't think it was helpful. She had married, was involved in a very conflictual relationship with her husband, had no children, and was a "loner" except for having one woman friend. Her job as switchboard operator was her one success and it seemed to keep her functioning in other areas.

The long-term history of this girl points up one of the pitfalls of labeling. The clinicians had described her in specific dynamic terms in childhood and their description seems to be appropriate even now when her social maladjustment in adulthood is rated moderately severe. The label "psychosis," however, had eventuated from having to give one name to her pathology and, at the time of the clinic contact, the flagrant disturbance in her thought processes had been the deciding factor. It now seems that "inadequate personality" might have been a more appropriate primary diagnosis, but this category is applied only to adults, not children.

It was the two other children who had also been diagnosed as psychotic in childhood whose outcomes were unexpectedly favorable. These two, Andy, who was 15 at referral, and Bill, who was 10, had some similarities in their presenting symptoms and personality characteristics and in the disequilibrium of their immediate families.

Both Andy and Bill were intellectually bright and both were extremely hostile toward their parents although they expressed anger in different ways. They came from families where conflict was continual and where mother played the son off against an inadequate, passive-aggressive father. Both boys were separated intermittently during childhood from their mothers for periods of months at a time. Andy's mother was hospitalized after he was 12 and she was diagnosed manic depressive with paranoid trends. Bill's mother and father were separated many times, divorced once when Bill was 3 years old, remarried when he was 5, and are now, at follow-up, divorced again. When parents were separated, Bill was "boarded out" so that mother could work. Both Andy and Bill were evaluated in the Clinic as "latently psychotic" and both exhibited fairly serious disruption of ego boundaries with paranoid and magical thinking in reference to the dangers they perceived in their environment.

Andy's ego disorganization had seemed to begin to occur only some 2 or 3 years prior to his referral at age 15. He had functioned well in school until he was in the 8th grade. Always a rebellious, assertive boy, Andy became almost unmanageable when father began to withdraw the attention he had always lavished on this son to favor, instead, Andy's older brother. Mother was hospitalized during this time. Then, at about 12 years of age, Andy began to have fits of rage when he seemed to be completely out of control as he screamed and hit at brother and parents.

The parents cited, as another precipitating event before Andy's dramatic change in personality, his finding his uncle dead. Andy had been very close to this uncle who lived with the family. The uncle, who was blind, died from loss of blood in an accident in the home.

At follow-up, Andy, 28 years old, was functioning very well. Although the parents had refused therapy at the Clinic, Andy had had a year and a half of outpatient therapy elsewhere. He had graduated from college, was employed in a managerial position and had been married for four years to a woman he described as "good for me—she can handle problems much better than I can." Andy lives in a state far from his parents to whom he no longer feels close emotionally. Interestingly, his first move out of his parents' house was to the formerly envied brother's house and he sees that move as very growth-producing. His college career was a satisfying experience both academically and socially.

Bill's childhood was more consistently pathological than Andy's. Bill had been shifted from one baby sitter to another while mother worked. His resentment was expressed in a way different from Andy's open hostility. He was brought to the Clinic because he had begun, at age 7, to soil his pants and to withdraw into a world of preoccupation with space, insects, and collections of various kinds. He turned his aggression toward himself. For example, under stressful conditions, he would hit himself repeatedly.

Bill was age 22 when interviewed at follow-up. He had just returned from 4 years of military service where he had done well in radar school and he was planning to go to college the next semester. He had also done well in high school and made a few close friendships which he has retained.

It seems that two experiences were especially important in Bill's dramatic improvement. He and his parents had undergone a long period of therapy at the Clinic. At first the parents and Bill were seen separately but when no change was evident after two years, it was decided that Bill's and the parents' therapist, working together, would see the three in family therapy. After another two years, therapy could be terminated with this family which was considered to have made "massive therapeutic change."

In addition to relief of his symptoms, a major personality change was noted in that Bill was able to "pull himself together as a person" by using the family sessions to "fill in the gaps" in his life when parents were married, divorced, and remarried. He was also able to relate to and identify with father. Even though parents were divorced again before follow-up, Bill has kept up a relationship with father.

The other salutory experience in Bill's life seems to have been his successful military service where he was provided the structure he had lacked in childhood and where he could turn his intellectual preoccupations to practical advantage.

Only one of the four children diagnosed as psychotic seems to have been "autistic" in childhood. Tom was and still is quite autistic in spite of his long history of therapy. His course is like that of the nonmute subgroup of children in the Kanner and Eisenberg (1955) study who were found, on follow-up, to be able to attend school but who retained in adolescence and young adulthood their isolation, their attraction to objects rather than to people, and a contact with reality which was still tenuous.

Bill, who was referred to the Clinic at the same age as was Tom, 7 years, also had autistic preoccupations but they seem, from the vantage point of hindsight, to have been a defense against intolerable anxiety and to have become useful, subsequently, in the service of life functioning.

Andy's "psychosis" appears, now, to have been a temporary, albeit severe, disturbance during a period of great turbulence and trauma while Wanda may, indeed, have been misdiagnosed in childhood.

Adult Outcome in Borderline Psychosis

The Clinic used a diagnosis of "borderline psychosis" for those children who presented many symptoms from among "fixed obsessions, bizarre fantasies, peculiar, unusual behavior, low frustration tolerance, emotional immaturity, unevenness of development, periodic impulse breakthrough, poor judgment, deficiencies of object relations, lack of tolerance for heightened stimulation, and, at the slightest provocation, withdrawal from reality" (Appendix A). The distinction of this category from that of psychosis is mainly one of degree in loss of contact with reality. The borderline child exhibits only intermittent loss of contact. The extent and seriousness of the borderline child's symptoms and behaviors and the *pan*-anxiety he suffers serve to differentiate him from the neurotic child and those with personality disorders.

Fifteen of the 200 children were given the diagnostic label borderline psychosis by the clinical conference and they represented a wide variety of symptom and dynamic configurations. In some children, impulsive, acting out behavior predominated while others were withdrawn and isolated; some displayed intense, incapacitating anxiety while others showed little affect of any kind; some did well in school while others were not achieving in spite of adequate intellectual ability. Structurally, ego functions ranged from moderately to severely impaired and superego ranged from lax to rigid and punitive.

The array of symptoms, behaviors, and degree of impairment has made the diagnosis "borderline" somewhat of a "wastebasket" category. Even the clinical ratings of the intensity of the disturbance showed some range: they covered the three steps from "moderate" through "severe" to "incapacitating." Most of the children (11 of the 15) were rated as severely disturbed, one as incapacitated, and three others as moderately disturbed.

Only 3 of the 15 children, or 20%, were diagnosed borderline by both the research psychiatrist and psychologist, rating independently and without knowledge of the conference diagnosis. The psychiatrist and psychologist both designated one other child neurotic and one "organic brain syndrome." Among all 30 diagnostic judgments by psychiatrist and psychologist on these 15 children who were all called borderline in the clinic conferences, psychosis of some kind was the most frequent (12) with neurosis (7), organic brain syndrome (6), personality disorder (3), and developmental deviation (2) following in that order. This variety of diagnoses reflects the many clinical pictures which the group displayed.

The outcome in social adjustment of these 15 children who had been labeled borderline at their clinical conferences was, on the average, the poorest of the nine diagnostic groups. Even in this group, however, most of the children were rated somewhat improved at follow-up (10 of the 15). Four other children had retained their severely maladjusted or incapacitated status and one child was rated more maladjusted. For four of these five children with poor outcomes, either the research psychologist or psychiatrist (3 cases) or both (1 case) had agreed with the conference diagnosis of borderline and for the other child both of these research clinicians had presented a diagnosis of organic brain syndrome. Moreover, the possibility of organicity was, in fact, repeatedly mentioned in this group of 15 children as a second diagnosis, a finding that may bear some relation to other research which shows that children originally called psychotic are often found, later, to have some evidence of organicity (Rutter et al., 1968).

The unfavorable prognosis for this combination of organic signs and borderline psychosis was clearly demonstrated in two of the children.

David, who is described in Chapter 5 to illustrate the importance of referral at a young age, is one of these children. As a young adult, he is still engaging in the wild, aggressive behavior which began in preschool years and required that he be hospitalized during adolescence.

The Clinic psychiatrist, noting David's perpetual motion, his very impulsive behavior, poor concentration, and deficient learning ability, had diagnosed his disorder as an organic brain syndrome. The decision of the psychologist, like that of the conference team when David was 6, was of a psychotic process, incipient in nature. The psychologist's dynamic formulation of David at age 6 conforms to the usual description for borderline psychosis:

Ego development has been severely impaired. This child has not yet withdrawn into a world of fantasy and unreality completely but, under stress, he regresses into a psychotic state and this is close to becoming permanent. Differentiation of self from environment is only minimal and he desperately needs treatment if any hope of avoiding psychosis is to be entertained.

This prediction has proved to be accurate and it seems, now, at followup, that David has "crossed the border" into psychosis. He is at home, incapacitated as far as any independent existence is concerned, and is often completely out of contact in his murderous rages.

The presence of an organic basis for borderline psychosis is even more likely in Harold's case. He was born prematurely, weighing only 3.5 pounds, was always hyperactive and accident-prone, and had a severe auditory-perceptual problem Although at age 10, his Full Scale Intelligence Quotient was 93, his subtest scores ranged all the way from the mental defective to the superior range. The diagnosis "brain syndrome" was made by both the psychiatrist and psychologist of the research staff.

At the clinical conference, however, although the probability of organic factors was acknowledged, the overall picture had seemed to warrant the diagnosis of "borderline psychotic child." The Clinic psychiatrist's description of Harold fits this classification:

The lack of a stable internal structure results in variable function with sudden loss of significant objects. During periods of integrated functions, he demonstrates a surprising capacity for relationship and accurate perception of the environment but direct impulse expression interrupts (this) . . . . Aggression, dependency needs and anxiety related to shifting (ego) boundaries appear to furnish the major source of conflict.

Harold was seen in individual psychotherapy for over a year at the Clinic while his parents were in group therapy. He was also referred for special education and both experiences seemed to be partially successful in inducing better impulse control and learning efficiency.

When interviewed at age 23, Harold was single and living at home. He had been working as a hospital janitor but depended on drugs and a protective and supportive mother to help him avoid hospitalization. Actually, he *had* been hospitalized for 10 days between the first and second follow-up contact after he had threatened to kill his father and then tried to commit suicide.

Harold's history had been one of constant trouble with aggression, often of a serious nature. He appeared still to be "borderline psychotic" at follow-up and required continuing psychiatric and parental supervision.

In contrast to these children who were and now, in young adulthood, are still very deviant, several other borderline children were equally disturbed but were found, on follow-up, to be functioning well. In fact, two such children earned the best possible social adjustment ratings at follow-up and lowered, thereby, the average maladjustment ratings of the borderline group. Both children had very poor starts in life, one apparently because of physiological problems that were severe from birth on, and the other from maternal neglect and finally desertion.

These children are striking exceptions to findings of this study which assign long-term importance to manifestations of severe problems early in life. In Sally's case it is easy to point to changes in her life circumstances which could have reversed the early pathological trends. Such circumstances are not apparent to account for Gary's remarkable improvement.

Sally's early history reads like a textbook description of what should not happen to a child in the first years of life. Sally was the eighth of eleven children in a very poor family. Both father and mother were irresponsible parents and father was out of work much of the time. There were days at a time when there was so little food in the house that Sally and her younger siblings went hungry while the older children ate what food there was. The children were left on their own a great deal and fought constantly.

When Sally's aunt and uncle came from another state to visit the family, Sally, who was then 3 years old, "latched on" to them and begged to go home with them. Sally's mother had no objection and Sally left the same day. She was extremely underweight, vomited frequently, and slept little at night. Sally had pulled all her hair out. She was very aggressive toward children and adults alike but she also cried a great deal and had multiple fears. Her speech was so poor that it was difficult to understand what she wanted and she would become extremely angry and frustrated when she was not understood.

During the two years between the time Sally came to live with her aunt and uncle and their first contact with the clinic, Sally had improved in some areas, especially in physical health and in overcoming sadness. She was still very restless and aggressive, especially toward children. She still roamed the house at night but with less and less frequency. At times she seemed to be in a "daze," not hearing when she was spoken to. During a temper tantrum, Sally would destroy household objects and her toys, seemingly without awareness of what she was doing. She wanted to be near her aunt all the time.

The aunt and uncle were simple, even-tempered people whose philosophy of raising children was that they needed a great deal of love, but also guidance and firmness. "If children are handled correctly, the need for firmness shouldn't be very much."

As might be expected from her early deprivation and trauma, Sally was found, in the Clinic's diagnostic study, to have inadequate ego structure for her age, a poor sense of her own identity, little impulse control, and a tenuous hold on reality. A host of neurotic symptoms and of antisocial tendencies plus these ego defects led to the diagnosis of borderline psychosis.

This child and her aunt were seen less than a dozen times in all with sessions at intervals of several months in a "supportive clinic" within the Clinic's program. The aunt was given advice as to how to cope with Sally's behavior and fears while Sally was seen merely on a relationship basis. Sally had a very good grade school experience with teachers who consulted with the Clinic regularly. Her progress there was slow but steady.

At follow-up, Sally presented the picture of quite an ordinary 18-year-old who was entering her senior year at high school and was achieving at the low-average level which was commensurate with her intellectual ability. She got along well with peers and teachers, participated in several school sports, and worked part time as an office helper at school. Sally was planning on a nursing career and had already arranged to begin working as a nurse's aid during the summer.

The spectacular improvement in this girl over a thirteen-year span can easily be attributed to the complete change in her family environment after age 3. She had had no other professional help after her few sessions at the Clinic. Her aunt recalled, in her follow-up interview, what a poor future the Clinic had predicted for Sally. The aunt had "just kept on trying," however. "I knew she could learn if I sat down with her and helped her."

One interesting speculation is that, in addition to the investment of "tender, loving care" on the part of the aunt and uncle, Sally had a major natural asset in her own assertive reaching out for help at age 3. She was, after all, the one child in her large family who got herself out of the deprived and unhealthful situation.

In contrast to Sally's impoverished background, Gary came from a family whose socioeconomic status was above average. Both parents were well-educated and talented. However, since father's occupation made it necessary for them to move often and for the parents to live apart most of the time, mother was responsible for most of the care of the children and experienced this as an extreme burden. Highly nervous herself, she found Gary's extreme irritability almost beyond her ability to handle. Gary had been a highstrung, colicky child from birth on. He suffered from projectile vomiting, slept little at night, and cried for hours at a time.

Problems at school started with his entrance and had continued unabated to the time he was referred to the Clinic at age 9. Teachers complained that he lied, stole, cheated, fought other children, and used vulgar language. They gave him credit for being a good leader although he often led his schoolmates in rebellion against the teachers.

The extent of Gary's pathology became evident in the clinical diagnostic evaluation. His overt aggressive behavior was accompanied, at the intrapsychic level, by intense despair over his inability to get dependency needs satisfied and "by feelings that he must take what he can get while always having to fear that he will be caught, punished, and destroyed for his attempts to get the love and attention he needs."

Gary displayed frequent regression to aggressive orality, reality testing was fluid, and ego boundaries were not always maintained. The diagnosis of borderline psychosis with pervasive anxiety was agreed upon in the conference and he was referred to a special school for emotionally disturbed children. The family soon moved again, however, and did not carry through on the Clinic's recommendation.

Gary's adjustment as a young adult was remarkable. He was in his second year of junior college and worked part time. Although he was a quiet, reserved person, he had several friends and was well-liked by his peers. He had had a steady girlfriend for nearly a year. Gary himself commented that he knew he had been a "real trouble maker as a kid" and blamed his mother for not having been strict enough with him. He remembered having to move around the country so much—"I would just make friends and then I had to leave them."

The follow-up interview revealed nothing tangible on which to base the change in Gary from ages 9 to 22. He had certainly had a poor start in life, especially in his physiological functioning, and there may have been some organic basis for his irritability. But other than the natural process of growing up and gradually establishing better ego control, nothing else appeared in the study from which to try to "explain" his improvement.

Adult Outcome of the Neurotic Children

The diagnosis of neurosis in childhood was, by far, the most frequently assigned at the clinical conference, with 100 children, or 50%, of the research sample so designated. There was, moreover, much better agreement among the research psychologist and psychiatrist and the clinical conference on this than on most of the other diagnoses. In contrast to the diagnosis of borderline psychosis where the research psychologist and psychiatrist agreed on that diagnosis in only 3 of the 15 (or 20%) cases so designated in clinical conference, the diagnosis of neurosis was the only one given to 59 of the 100 conference-diagnosed neurotic children and another 28 of them were called neurotic by one of the two research diagnosticians.

It seems that whereas the poor agreement for the "borderline" diagnosis may result from the variety of symptom and behavior patterns to which this diagnosis was applied in conference, it may be easier to agree upon the two main characteristics of neurosis: the presense of anxiety and an intact ego. Of the 41 conference-labeled neurotic children on which there was disagreement from the research professionals, 6 were called *neurotic* behavior disorders by at least one of the two judges, a diagnosis which, like that of neurosis, indicates the presence of anxiety.

The wide difference between the neurotic and psychotic designation is supported by the fact that of these 100 children labeled neurotic at the conference, only one was called psychotic by both the psychiatrist and psychologist of the research staff and this subject was indeed extraordinary. (The history of this girl who was unexpectedly rated "healthy" in adjustment at follow-up is reviewed later.) For another 5 of the 100 neurotic children, one of the two research professionals offered a diagnosis of psychosis. The majority of the 41 children on whom there was disagreement were thought by the research professionals to have some kind of personality disorder in childhood.

As is true in the reports of most other follow-up studies, the majority of the neurotic children in this study had favorable outcomes in adulthood. Fifty-six of the 100 were rated healthy or only mildly maladjusted in social functioning as young adults, 27 showed moderate maladjustment, 16 were considered to be severely disturbed, and only one was "incapacitated."

Two patterns emerge among these latter 17 children who turned out severely maladjusted. One was that of the depressed neurotic child. Eight of the 17 were labeled "depressed" by one or both of the research diagnosticians. The other pattern includes those children called neurotic at the conference but classed as "oppositional," "isolated," or "impulse-ridden" personality disorders by one or both researchers (6 of the 17 children). The *only* neurotic child to be classified incapacitated in adulthood was judged by both research diagnosticians to be depressed in childhood. (Her history is reviewed in Chapter 5 under the pseudonym "Marilyn.") Some of the other depressed children were rated as very maladjusted in adulthood but not incapacitated.

Rosalie has been weighted down by a heavy burden of depression throughout her young life. She was crying when her mother first brought her to the Clinic at age 6 and she continued to cry through most of the diagnostic process. She was reported to have suffered extreme separation anxiety when she first started to school and intermittently thereafter throughout grade and high school. The clinical picture was that of a classic "school phobia" with a very hostile-dependent relationship to mother who unconsciously encouraged the interaction while overtly resenting Rosalie's clinging to her.

Unable to express her hostility directly, Rosalie had turned much of it against herself. She was often "sick at her stomach"; at school she had become the victim of other children's teasing. Her projective tests revealed a self-concept of badness and damage in spite of her strict morals and good intellectual assets. Rosalie had many other fears in addition to that of going to school. Some of them interfered markedly with her peer relationships for example, her fear of visiting at other children's houses. She spent almost all her free time at home with her mother and sister.

Rosalie presented a pathetic picture when interviewed at follow-up. She had finished high school after several occasions of "dropping out" and was enrolled in her freshman year of college. She told a plaintive story of repeated disappointments and continual unhappiness. She had no friends at all outside her family circle. Her only companion near her own age was her sister who, according to Rosalie, "feels sorry for me now and then and takes me along with her." Rosalie had had only a couple of dates and these were "blind dates" arranged by her sister. She works part time as a bookkeeper, an occupation she describes thus: "It's just a job— not what I'd like to do. I just sit back there in the office all by myself— sometimes one of the bosses comes in to complain to me when he's bored." Rosalie spends her evenings watching television, mainly in her own room.

Rosalie has been in therapy on several occasions and with several psychiatrists since she had her diagnostic workup at the Clinic. She found it very difficult to talk to her therapists and felt that only one of them had helped her. "It was when I was going to try to go back to high school after I had been out a whole year. I was so afraid and I needed help. He was a wonderful psychiatrist but I couldn't talk much even to him so he had me keep a diary all week and bring it in. But after a short time, he and his wife had a baby and they moved to another state. I still wrote to him."

Mother is painfully aware of Rosalie's unhappiness. As she walked with the interviewers to their car, the mother summarized her impression of her daughter's life experience: "I watched her miss her childhood, then her adolescence and now that she is an adult, she is still barely existing."

Rosalie is an extreme example of a group of neurotic children whose disturbance was obviously *not* temporary and whose behavior has remained self-defeating and anxiety-laden. In her case the pathological relationship to her mother was and seems to be still at the root of her illness. While she has suffered little ego disorganization, Rosalie is indeed a severely disturbed young adult both socially and internally.

The child who is neurotically depressed does not always continue the same kind of anxious, fearful, and depressed syndrome into adulthood as did Rosalie. The overt behavior of several of the other depressed children was found, at follow-up, to be antisocial, even delinquent. In some cases this trend toward delinquency was noted even in childhood although the more observable pathology had been pervasive depression.

Ted was an unwanted child, the eldest of three in a family in which mother wanted to work outside the home and father assumed little responsibility for the children. Ted was tended by one baby-sitter after another. Mother, a dominant but dissatisfied woman, resented father's passivity but realized, also, that she could not have lived with a more aggressive man. Actually, the couple was apart during much of Ted's early childhood with father working out of town.

During their first Clinic contact, when Ted was 10, mother had nothing positive to say about her only son. She lumped him, her husband, and her father together as exceedingly lazy, selfish, and stubborn males. Mother talked openly in her first interview at the Clinic about her wish to be rid of Ted—"If I never saw him again that would be just fine. It's terrible to feel that way about your own child but that's exactly the way I feel."

Much of the actual behavior that mother resented so much was of a passively hostile nature such as shutting out mother's critical tirades or seeming to comply but actually doing what he wanted to do. His misbehaviors were largely petty misdeeds such as lying to get out of trouble, failing to keep promises and to "follow rules." Even though mother thought of Ted as "the bad seed," she was aware of his general unhappiness and his feeling unloved and rejected both at home and among his peers.

The Clinic's diagnostic team concurred in a diagnosis of neurotic depression and this was the independently made decision of the research psychologist and psychiatrist who reviewed the clinical material. Ted's passive-aggressive behavior was seen as an ineffective, defensive maneuver against feelings of extreme worthlessness. His projective test productions contained suicidal themes. Although he revealed strong impulses to act out, he generally found this behavior too threatening and turned his aggression toward himself. What acting out he did was likely to be of a sneaking, undercover kind to insure his safety from authority figures whom he feared. His failure to produce at school seemed to be part of this "play-safe" strategy.

The parents had a difficult time accepting any responsibility for Ted's problems. They failed to complete the diagnostic process on their first Clinic contact but returned two years later to report that Ted was "totally miserable" and had to have help. Although they insisted that they were now ready to go through with the diagnostic evaluation and follow the Clinic's recommendations, mother dropped out of her own casework process after a few sessions and took Ted out of group therapy, against advice, at the end of the first year.

In the group, Ted started out as a compliant, passive "good guy" who constantly tried to please the therapist. He gradually became more assertive and more able to express hostility directly. His therapist recorded that he did not believe Ted had made much progress. However, he had been able to relate to the other boys in the group and begin to make a masculine identification with the therapist.

Ted was 23 at follow-up interview. His affect during the interview seemed bland rather than depressed but he said he does get depressed over his inability to make or keep friends. He described himself as a "loner" but he has been in trouble with the law several times as part of a gang of boys who drink and stay out all night. He has been arrested and jailed for destroying property. He has difficulty in keeping a job, mainly because he has to "tell the boss off."

Ted's relationship with his family is very poor. He is overly involved with his mother in a mutually seductive relationship but she has evicted him several times when he has refused to get a job. Ted has special difficulty in relating to girls. "I don't want to get emotionally involved with any of them." Mother feels that Ted thinks the world owes him a living but that he also believes he really isn't deserving of anything.

Most of the 100 children who were diagnosed neurotic at the Clinic conference improved in adult social adjustment ratings even when their childhood maladjustment was rated "severe." (There were no ratings of "5," or incapacitated, among the neurotic children.) Of the 31 severely maladjusted (rated 4) neurotics, 25, or 81%, had improved in adulthood and only 6 were still severely maladjusted. One of those showing remarkable improvement is the one child who was judged by both research diagnosticians to have been borderline psychotic in childhood and had been called "severely neurotic with psychotic potential" at the Clinic conference.

Joanne was referred to the Clinic at age 9 when she refused to go to school. The eldest of five children, she was a bright, overly conscientious, rather compulsive child who was finding it impossible to satisfy a very strict teacher and to meet her own ideals for perfection in her schoolwork. The Clinic interviews revealed that mother and Joanne had been locked in a head-on struggle from infancy on. Joanne had resisted mother's attempts to control her at every turn and mother had retaliated with open censure and rejection, for example, "You are no good and never will be."

Except for the very strict teacher, Joanne got along with most of her teachers in the Catholic school she attended even though she periodically refused to go and was especially resistant to attending daily Mass because she became afraid there.

Joanne's relationship to father was less conflicted than that with mother but he was a very passive man who had little to do with the discipline of Joanne and the other four children. Mother had felt very guilty over not wanting her first pregnancy so soon after marriage and for having had to leave Joanne several times during her first few years. These separations occurred when mother was hospitalized for childbirth, miscarriages, and operations. Mother had also suffered an extended postpartum depression after Joanne's birth.

It was in the Clinic evaluation that the extent and depth of Joanne's pathology was uncovered. Her fears about going to school and to church were seen, in the psychiatric and psychological diagnostic sessions, to be part of an intense fear of destruction brought on by guilt over the hostility she had for her mother. She had not made a feminine identification nor had she differentiated sexual roles in others.

Her boundaries between reality and fantasy were equally obscure. Her fantasy was clearly distorted by religious beliefs which she seemed to be using as justification for her refusal to accept her femininity. Both the Clinic psychiatrist and psychologist commented on the breakthrough of psychotic material; the diagnosis of "neurosis" at the conference was qualified with the impression of potential psychotic breakdown. Both research diagnosticians, working from the Clinic records, called her "borderline psychotic."

Inpatient treatment was recommended. After an initial reaction of shock at this extreme recommendation, the parents followed through and Joanne spent the next four years in a residential treatment center. She recalls thinking she must be "crazy" too when she first went to the center and saw what she thought were "crazy" children there. Now, she has fond memories of her experience at the center and thinks it made the difference in her life.

It is not surprising that Joanne chose the religious life as her career but what is surprising is the degree of improvement in life adjustment. She was seen twice for follow-up, first at age 23 and again at 25 for a more intensive evaluation by another interviewer. Both interviewers rated her overall adjustment at the "best" level (1) and both judged her relationships and functioning to be very good to excellent. Her improvement seems to have been continuous since her placement in the residential treatment center with increasingly good academic perform-ance, more participation in group activities, and better relationships with peers and authority figures.

She teaches school now and loves her work. She is regarded as a leader among the sisters in her community setting who apparently enjoy her sense of humor and her willingness to listen to their troubles. It is significant, of course, that Joanne has been able to continue her avoidance of sexuality through her choice of a vocation and equally significant that she chose the very line of work, teaching, from which her troubles stemmed in childhood. She seems, however, to be able to use her own bad experiences of childhood to benefit children under her care in a healthy, nondestructive way.

Joanne has sought therapeutic help a few times for short periods when confronted with some change in her life situation. It is a tribute to her early therapeutic experience that she has been aware of her need for outside help and has used it most effectively. She apparently defends against remnants of her early depression through work and group activity.

Neurotic Behavior Disorders vs. Character Disorders

Viewed from the standpoint of outcome, the Clinic's use of the category of "neurotic behavior disorder" in addition to those of "neurotic reaction" and "character disorder" was well-advised. The diagnostic manual reserved the first term for those reactions in which there was "significant admixture of ex-ternal and internalized conflict with some indication that guilt and/or anxiety is present . . ." and in which "there appears to be potential for reversing the re-gression that has taken place."

In the character disorder, on the other hand, "anxiety is minimized or ab-sent and anxiety occurs only in the face of punishment. . . . It very often reflects lifelong interpersonal conflict manifested as habitual, standardized and in-flexible modes of response" (Appendix A). This, the Clinic's definition of character disorder, was adopted from the descriptions of adult disorders and is probably too severe to be applied to children. The Clinic practice seems to have been to weigh the absence or degree of anxiety present and the intransigency of the maladaptive behavior patterns in deciding on one or the other diagnosis.

Twenty-four of the 200 children were labeled "neurotic behavior disorders" and 30 were called "character disorders" at their Clinic conferences. The average adult social adjustment rating of the former children was significantly better than that of those labeled character disorder.

The difference in outcome between the two groups of children is best illustrated, however, in the adult adjustment ratings of those in each category who were rated severe, or "4," in social maladjustment in childhood. Of the 8 children whose neurotic behavior disorders were rated severe, 5, or 62%, were found at follow-up to be well or only mildly maladjusted socially, while of the 15 childhood character disorders also rated 4 (severe), only 27% were in these two best categories of social adjustment. Thus, it seems that even if behavior manifestations are severe enough to earn a poor rating in childhood adjustment, the presence of clinically observable anxiety predicts a better chance for future life adjustment.

This type of child may improve even after a long history of rather serious behavior problems.

Larry had been a behavior problem at school for most of the six years prior to his referral to the Clinic at age 12. He was about to be suspended again for disobedience and resistance toward his 7th grade teacher, his cruelty toward other children, and his refusal to do the work assigned. Yet he tested in the superior range intellectually and placed in the 9th grade level on achievement tests. Mother excused Larry's behavior on the basis of his general unhappiness and insecurity. He resented never having had a father in the home; mother, by her own admission, was not strict enough in her discipline. Mother would even excuse the physical abuse she suffered at Larry's hands, seeing it as punishment due her for having given birth to him and his twin sister outside marriage.

Several relatives had helped now and then in the care of the two children but most of the time mother had to struggle with problems of keeping baby sitters while she worked. Larry's anger seemed to be directed especially toward his mother and sister and to have generalized to women teachers. He reached out for a relationship with male father figures, especially one financially successful uncle who was his ideal.

The Clinic recognized the seriousness of Larry's acting out behavior but sensed deep anxiety and depression behind his aggressive bravado. He seemed to be confused and very sad over the loss of the father he had never known. The clinical team thought Larry had the assets to benefit from psychotherapy but recommended that he be placed out of the home in a residential center where the opportunity for male identification and supervision as well as for therapy would be provided. Larry refused absolutely to accept placement. He went to live, for a time, with his aunt and uncle where his school and social adjustment improved temporarily.

During adolescence Larry was arrested for peace disturbance while under the influence of drugs. He dropped out of high school in the 11th grade but later passed the GED tests and enrolled in college courses at night school.

Larry's major improvement in functioning seems to have occurred in the four years before he was seen for follow-up at age 24. It is difficult to pinpoint the bases for the change, but, according to Larry, it was his own realization that he was heading into serious trouble and he had better "shape up." He took on -the-job training as a manufacturer's sales representative and has had several promotions in that occupation. He also gives credit to his wife, whom he met at age 19 and married a year later. She seems to be a very stable person to whom Larry can relate on a collateral level. "We are each other's best friend." They have bought their own home in a very nice suburban area.

Larry seems to be accomplishing many of the goals he had set for himself as a result of his admiration for his uncle. He is still somewhat anxious and his change toward socially acceptable behavior is still largely based on his need to succeed and to avoid punishment. One wonders if he will be able to maintain his new way of life if misfortune should enter in. He feels confident in his ability to do so.

The probability that there will be a decided change in antisocial behavior is much less when it is accompanied by few inner resources and little anxiety.

Like Larry, Louis was considered by his family always to have been an "angry child." He simply would not mind. "Father would spank him and put him in a corner, but he would come out and do the same thing again and get spanked again." Both parents were extremely strict. They had come from deprived backgrounds and wanted their children to grow up to be "good citizens" and have a different life than they had had. Mother, who had been beaten by her father many times, felt some obligation to protect Louis when his father lost control in punishing him.

Louis was particularly fatalistic in his attitude toward his problems when he came to the Clinic at age 15. He was aware of his lack of impulse control but had little hope of gaining control through his parents' way of "handling" him. He could envision only further antisocial behavior and eventual destruction of himself. He was unable to identify with a father whom he saw as passive and ineffectual but potentially destructive.

Louis was one of the older subjects seen in the follow-up. At 28, he was an unemployed truck driver. He had been fired for physically attacking his boss, an attack which he felt was justified because the boss was "unfair" to him. He had been discharged from military service a few years earlier as "incapable of adapting to military life."

His relationship to his family was still a hostile, dependent one. He and his father argued constantly. "Sometimes I don't talk to dad or mom at all for weeks at a time." His relationship with peers is equally poor. He described much rowdy, antisocial behavior with a gang of fellows who rode motorcycles in a group. "I used to get so smacked when I was out with them that the guys would put me on my cycle and head me toward my house." He is proud of his marksmanship with a gun. "I keep a pistol and it's loaded. Dad ordered me to get rid of it but I wouldn't."

Louis' need to prove his masculinity in these symbolic ways is accompanied by an intense hatred of homosexual men. "I can't tolerate bisexual men and if I meet one in a dark alley, I'll smack them up. If they want their teeth, they'd better keep moving." Louis' ambivalence about heterosexuality is clear and his attempts to relate to females has been extremely disappointing. "I just drop girls without even calling them up. I don't trust them. I try to carry on longer with them but I just can't." Louis spends his leisure time with "the boys," at singles dances or at an archery range.

Louis has seen two psychiatrists since he was at the Clinic where he had only the diagnostic. He was referred for psychiatric help after acting out while in the military service and again more recently. He dismissed these therapeutic contacts with the statement: "I was told that I am an angry person and I've decided that I really am."

The consistent, unchanging course of Louis' antisocial behavior seems singularly unrelated to any internal process of learning from experience, let alone to internal anxiety. He does become depressed and pessimistic over his belief that his hostility will lead, eventually, to his destruction.

Although the majority of children whose social adjustment was rated as severely deviant and who were clinically diagnosed as "character disorders" were found, at follow-up, still to be severely maladjusted in life functioning, there were a few surprising exceptions to this finding. Of 15 severely maladjusted children in the character disorder group, four have made adequate young adult adjustments. Moreover, there was a wide variety in the amount of intervention within these four cases, from no treatment at all in the case of one child, to a heavy expenditure of both outpatient and residential treatment over a period of years in another case.

At age 14½, Shirley presented a classic picture of an hysterical character disorder. She was described by her mother and stepfather as "extremely hard to handle, unreasonable and rebellious, antagonistic and stubborn. She seems to feel the whole family is there just for her benefit." Her acting out behavior was largely sexual in nature. She was extremely seductive, and the stepfather, a reformed alcoholic, unable to resist her sexual attractiveness, repeatedly made sexual advances toward her.

Shirley's mother had several nervous breakdowns and was hospitalized for these and for accidental injuries. Early in life, Shirley had to be placed in an "orphanage" because of mother's illnesses.

The intensive diagnostic study at the Clinic found little in the way of anxiety in Shirley's dynamics. She felt she had been rejected by natural father and by mother and that she was entitled to grab whatever happiness she could out of life. She used her superior intellectual ability and her good looks to manipulate others into giving to her as one would to an appealing, needful child.

Shirley added much color to the group therapy sessions in which she participated for about two years. She entered the group in a breezy, sophisticated manner and promptly tried to shock the other girls with tales of daring behavior and sexual exploits. While these accounts were probably highly exaggerated, she had been acting out enough that her stepfather decided, after one of her escapades, that she could not live in his house another day and proceeded to "dump" her bodily at the Clinic. No amount of persuasion from the therapist could change the stepfather's decision to get rid of Shirley.

In the family session set up to discuss the emergency situation, Shirley blandly announced that she knew she was "bad," that she had had to make up her mind whether she would be good or bad, and she just couldn't find any reason to be good. Moreover, the kids she was going around with were having too much fun being bad.

Shirley had to be placed that same day, first, on an emergency basis, in the detention home and a few days later in a girls' home where she stayed for nearly four years. She continued in group therapy during part of this time and seemed to make a relationship of a superficial kind with the other girls and, finally, a dependent relationship to the therapist. She was quite capable of "insight" of a logical type. A year after she had dropped out of the group, she returned to tell the therapist, "I *knew* what my troubles were and where they came from. It was just that I *had* to go ahead and get into trouble—I couldn't stop myself."

The troubles she got into were many. She struck up an acquaintance with a very irresponsible soldier who was AWOL, married him at 18 when she found she was pregnant, and lived with him on and off for several years. He spent much time in the army psychiatric hospital while she worked to support their two children. The husband beat Shirley and it was only when his physical abuse caused her to miscarry their third child that she had the courage to leave him for good. There followed several years in which Shirley worked and cared for the two children. This was apparently a period in which she "got her head together" and found out she could be a capable, reliable worker and a good mother on her own.

At follow-up, Shirley was married again, this time to an apparently mature, responsible man who seemed to care a great deal for her and the children, including one born of this, Shirley's second marriage. She told the interviewer that she attributed her change in functioning to the therapy she had at the Clinic and to the residential center which she called "home." She still has frightening dreams about her experiences in early life and in adolescence. "Without the Clinic, I wouldn't be here today."

In the Clinic chart the closing summary by Shirley's therapist contains this prediction: "In spite of Shirley's breaking treatment and marrying a disturbed and irresponsible young man, it is felt that she gained enough in treatment that she will be able to use this help after her present turmoil is over. She was able to make some superficial gains and had it not been for the turmoil of adolescence she might have made deeper gains."

Another child with a serious characterological disorder in childhood has also made a satisfactory adjustment but without the formal therapeutic intervention afforded Shirley. This kind of history distorts the statistical findings of outcome that are expected for this particular diagnostic group.

Scott was left with his aunt right after birth because mother was unmarried and had no way to support him. He was raised by this aunt and another aunt in a domestic situation where one of them served as the strict, wage-earning father and the other as a giving, permissive mother. In addition, Scott was visited now and then by natural mother and, separately, by father, both of whom let him know he was their son. The Clinic social worker, after interviewing the aunts for intake, commented in her report on the close, binding relationship between the boy and his fatherly aunt—"she sleeps with the boy and she beats him."

By the time he was referred by the school counselor to the Clinic when he was 7, Scott was extremely hyperactive and so constantly disruptive in the classroom that he had been suspended from school on many occasions. Although likeable in many respects, he was impulsive and manipulative. As might be expected, Scott had great difficulty in knowing who he was, whom to relate to as a parent, and what a male should be like and act like. The Clinic recognized the extent and seriousness of these problems but simply had no good solutions to offer. After their diagnostic study the staff concluded: "The situation in the home is such that it will continue to be detrimental to Scott and there are no practical solutions available for him such as removing him from the home."

The Clinic social worker did make several practical suggestions, however, that may have made a real difference in Scott's adjustment. These included less closeness, that is, seductiveness, in the relationship to his aunt with an outright request that she get the boy his own bed and, hopefully, his own bedroom. The aunt soon provided both without the expected resistance or difficulty. Also recommended was that Scott take part in boys' groups where a male leader was available and the aunt immediately took steps to have him included in a boys' club at a nearby church with a young minister as leader. It seemed that Scott's aunt could accept concrete advice and act on it at once.

When seen for the research at age 19, Scott was in junior college where he had a solid average grade record, was employed part time, and was helping his aunt with part of his school expenses. He had developed an interest in sports in high school and was on the basketball and football teams. He described very simple and realistic goals for himself such as to pass all his courses, to play well, and to get a car. He is achieving all these, including the last one.

Scott has many friends, both male and female. He dates regularly but tries not to get too serious with any one girl. All in all, his aunt is very satisfied with Scott's behavior. Scott commented, "She says she hasn't had any trouble with me so I guess I'm doing all right."

Throughout the years, the aunt has encouraged Scott to keep in touch with both natural parents. He goes to visit each of them. His aunt "demands" that Scott respect his parents "since they *are* his parents even if they still haven't grown up."

After a rocky early childhood, Scott seems to have settled down under the strict control of an aunt who has cared for him in her own way and who has defined limits and expectations clearly. He has made a masculine indentification in spite of his female environment and can also relate to the opposite sex. It is impossible to know, of course, what part, if any, the Clinic's diagnostic process and concrete "guidance" played in the change in Scott's life history.

The "Incapacitated" Children and the "Incapacitated" Adults

One of the foremost goals of research such as this is to trace the continuity of severe pathology in the hope that serious illness in adulthood may eventually be prevented or ameliorated by intervention in childhood. This study affords the opportunity 1) to look closely at those children who were considered to be seriously maladjusted already in childhood and to follow this adjustment into adulthood and 2) to reconsider the childhood characteristics of those young adults who were seriously maladjusted at follow-up. The children and young adults who were considered to be "incapacitated" in social functioning (rated 5) are a select portion of those subjects who were seriously disturbed at one or the other point in time.

In contrast to several other follow-up studies, the outpatient child guidance sample used in this research did not include many extremely maladjusted children and the exclusion of retarded children further limited the number who were incapacitated socially. In fact, only one child of the 200 studied was so designated and he was also one of the four individuals found to be socially incapacitated at follow-up. This boy's history is reviewed in Chapter 5 under the pseudonym "David."

David's antisocial, extremely destructive behavior was part of a life-long disturbance diagnosed as "borderline psychotic" and it has seemed to continue on into young adulthood with little change. Intervention in David's case had consisted of early placement in a children's home and forced hospitalization in a state hospital at age 14. It seems from the history that the early onset of his extreme and pervasive pathology and his inability to use environmental change to his advantage are factors in his lack of improvement.

In addition to David, the other three young adults who were judged, at follow-up, to be incapacitated were one other boy who was also diagnosed borderline psychotic in childhood, one diagnosed character disorder, and "Marilyn" who was first diagnosed severely neurotic and later borderline psychotic. Her history is also reviewed in Chapter 5.

Marilyn deteriorated rapidly in early adolescence soon after referral to the Clinic. Ego structure was probably brittle from early childhood on. She was described as a "model child" in grade school, overly compliant at home, and industrious at school. After one stormy period of a few months in early adolescence, Marilyn began to withdraw into a shell from which she has never completely emerged. Her history is reminiscent of Anna Freud's description of the adolescent who takes one look at the conflict and regression which adolescence normally entails and withdraws from it into his own, more manageable inner world.

The other two children, both boys, had exhibited serious problems from a very early age. Both were referred to the Clinic for school failure accompanied by troublesome classroom behavior which, in the case of Ralph, had begun at age 6 and had become so extreme that he had been expelled from school for a year before referral to child guidance at age 14.

Both boys had birth and neonatal histories suggestive of organic damage and, in Ralph's case, an electroencephalogram at age 8 supported this probability. He often went completely out of control during a temper tantrum and his behavior during these incidents was described as "psychotic-like." Mother and stepfather were unable to cope with him and, at age 8, he was placed in a residential children's center. When referred by this center to the Clinic for a diagnostic study at age 14, he was judged to be schizoid and so severely disturbed that he should be moved to an inpatient hospital setting.

At follow-up at age 26, Ralph was living in a "half-way house" maintained by the state hospital to rehabilitate former patients. He has spent most of his life in institutions including the children's home, the state hospital, and the state prison. He had never been able to keep a job and his arrest and conviction were for burglary. Ralph is still a "loner" whose only friends are a few people he met while he was in the hospital. He doesn't go out with girls and doesn't plan to marry unless, he says, he might meet a "rich old lady."

This history obviously depicts a continuous sequence of pathological factors, in constitutional makeup and in environmental circumstances. He was physically ill at birth and was rejected even before birth by mother who perceived him as being "born evil" like his "evil" father. Mother was happy to have him placed away from her in institutions and, even now, is worried that he may return home to become a burden to her.

It is difficult to imagine what kind of intervention other than those he experienced might have "saved" this child. Perhaps he could have benefited from some kind of special foster home in the very beginning to provide the unusual care that his physical and psychological illness warranted. Certainly he entered the first grade with behavior patterns already established that were bound to alienate him from teachers and classmates and to interfere with learning to a degree that eventuated in school failure. It was apparently already late by the time he was 8 to provide much help for Ralph.

The fourth incapacitated young adult, Warren, had returned home, at age 23, to live with his parents after his marriage of four years had ended in divorce. Both he and his wife had become drug addicts and he had been hospitalized several times for treatment of addiction. His only friends at present are "old dope buddies." He hasn't worked in years and usually spends his time in his room or "out in the woods." The parents are afraid of Warren and don't want him at home but have been unsuccessful in efforts to get the courts to recommit him.

Warren's childhood misbehavior was not as extreme nor parental rejection as absolute as that of Ralph. Warren's intellectual ability was only dull normal and required his placement in special classes throughout his school career. He dropped out in 10th grade to get a job. Warren's limited resources were undoubtedly a factor in some of his difficulties. He was highly suggestible, showed poor judgment, and was accident-prone.

His problems became serious in his middle teens. Mother dated their onset at age 17 when Warren bought an old car. He began running around with the town's most undesirable characters, started using hard drugs, and then married a girl who, apparently, was also disturbed. His mother now refers to her son as "a mess, a hopeless wreck who doesn't want to help himself." The parents have to keep drugs and guns away from him for fear he may harm himself or others, especially father whom Warren hates.

This boy was not considered to be extremely disturbed at the time of the Clinic's diagnostic evaluation when he was 12. He was diagnosed then as having a severe passive-aggressive personality disorder. His intellectual dullness and his inability to handle aggression except through counterphobic defenses which proved harmful to himself were noted and the parents and Warren were offered treatment in the Clinic's supportive unit. They continued in this "guidance" approach for two years with sessions at intervals of 2 to 4 weeks. When treatment was terminated by mutual agreement, Warren seemed, according to the Clinic record, "to be doing adequately in most ways."

Apparently Warren became disorganized when the stress of adolescence was more than his weak and suggestible ego could handle. His course after dropping out of school has been all downhill. It may be that the full extent of his intrapsychic disturbance was not recognized in childhood and/or that he could have benefited from more intensive therapy. In any case, his chances for making permanent use of the therapeutic and environmental help he was afforded seem to have been limited, probably by constitutional, and especially intellectual, inferiority.

These descriptions of children who did or did not conform to the outcome expected for the diagnostic category to which they had been assigned in childhood reflect the wide diversity in personality patterns, familial relationships, and social adaptation within any category. This diversity is a core problem in diagnosis and in prediction. When the follow-up data for a particular child can be integrated with a backward look at his early characteristics and life history, it is often possible to understand his adult adjustment more clearly than is possible from the analysis of group data alone.

CHAPTER 7

Treatment As Related To Outcome

A major question regarding the efficacy of treatment arose from the findings of this study. Why was it that untreated children obtained significantly healthier adult adjustment ratings than treated children? Most research points to comparable outcome of treated and untreated groups, especially for neurotic children.

Taken at face value, the findings of this study suggested that children obtain somewhat better outcome ratings if left untreated, rather than treated. The data were further examined to obtain plausible explanations for the findings. Areas considered included variables related to the treatment experience, children's recall of their clinic experience, comparability of the subjects and their families, and the basis for selection of children for treatment.

TREATMENT VARIABLES

Data were obtained on a few variables related to treatment: therapist's experience, length and type of therapy, number of therapists, and involvement of one or both parents in treatment. Parental involvement and type of therapy were not related to outcome. However, the quality of parental involvement is not known and effectiveness of the work with parents was not assessed.

The only therapist variable considered was that of experience as determined by the therapist's status as trainee or staff member, but this proved to be a fairly strong factor. Staff members were experienced clinicians—psychiatrists and psychologists—who carried training as well as direct service responsibilities in the clinic. Trainees were in training as psychologists or psychiatrists. The psychology interns were Ph.D. candidates with considerable academic background but little clinical experience, while the psychiatric residents had completed several years of training in adult psychiatry but were inexperienced in child therapy.

Those children treated by an experienced clinician as compared to a trainee obtained significantly healthier adult ratings. Furthermore, when adult outcome ratings of staff-treated children were compared with those of untreated children, differences in outcome were not significant. Both staff-treated and untreated children were below the total sample mean for adult outcome. Thus, it is evident that the treatment provided by inexperienced therapists accounted, to a considerable extent, for the difference in outcome ratings of treated and untreated children (see Table 22).

Now the question arises: Were staff-treated children less disturbed than those treated by trainees? On two measures that had significant correlations with adult outcome for the total sample, intensity of disturbance and diagnosis, the staff- and trainee-treated children did not differ.

Relatively little attention has been given in other research to the effects on outcome of therapist variables such as experience, personality characteristics, and theoretical orientation. As to the factor of experience, findings are varied. For example, Brown (1960), Levitt (1963), and Love and Kaswan (1974) found no significant differences in therapists' experience in relation to outcome whereas Cartwright and Vogel (1960) found more favorable outcome with experienced than inexperienced therapists. The inconsistency in findings among different studies suggests that the effect of experience may be compounded by other important variables.

Studies of therapists' personality characteristics, techniques, or approaches primarily with adult patients, suggest that such qualities as warmth, acceptance, empathy, and sensitivity are related to outcome (Rutter, 1975). Ricks (1974), in studying two therapists' work with 28 fairly disturbed adolescent boys, found that their different approaches led to different outcomes. Therapist A had positive results with an ego-supportive approach focused on immediate problems. With a comparable group of boys, therpaist B had less positive results with an anxiety-producing approach focused on unconscious repressed material. Thus, for this particular kind of adolescent, the specific approach was related to outcome.

Findings are varied as to the relationship of length of treatment to outcome. In the present research there was a trend toward better outcome with longer treatment as was also found in David's (1976) study of very disturbed children. Levitt (1971), in his review of child therapy research, did not find evidence of a relationship between length of treatment and outcome, while Lessing (1966) indicated such a relationship but questioned the independence of treatment

Table 22.   Relationship of Outcome in Clinic-Treated Children to Experience of Therapist

Treatment	N = 103	Mean Adult Adjustment[*]
Experienced staff	29	9.76
Inexperienced trainee	17	12.47
Both staff and trainee	7	9.71
Untreated	50	8.76

[*]$F = 5.429$, $p < .002$.

length and outcome measures. He drew attention to the fact that treatment may be terminated because those being treated were not making progress or were resistant and withdrew, or because treatment was completed.

Studies of brief treatment make a case for the efficiency and effectiveness of such therapy, suggesting that it is as good as long term, can service more people, and is more efficient. Rosenthal and Levine (1970) report a study of brief treatment in which both the therapeutic approach and the time factor differed from traditional long-term approaches. In their study, the average length of brief treatment was 8.1 weeks and that of long-term treatment was 39.9 weeks. Although they suggested that improvement rates were comparable in the two groups, this conclusion was not substantiated by the data. Fifty-five percent of the brief treatment cases and 79% of the long-term cases improved.

Leventhal and Weinberger (1975) reported a large scale study of brief therapy but did not compare it with long-term except to indicate that fewer families withdrew from brief than from long-term therapy. The average number of interviews per family in their study was 13.7 in brief therapy as contrasted with 38 in long-term, thus, the claim for greater efficiency; of the brief treatment cases, 61% improved, a proportion comparable to the 66% reported by Levitt (1971) in his review of therapy outcome research.

In the present study children treated by more than one therapist had better outcome ratings than those treated by one therapist. Although the two or more therapist cases were of significantly longer duration than those with one therapist, they also included children who were treated by a trainee followed by a staff therapist. It is possible that the outcome of two-therapist cases was confounded by treatment length and therapist experience as well as other variables not assessed. The small number of cases involved precludes a definitive conclusion regarding these issues.

This review of therapy variables suggests that some of them, notably therapist's experience, length of treatment, and number of therapists, should be explored further with appropriate control of these variables and analysis of both their separate and combined effects on outcome.

A final factor of potential relevance in the evaluation of the effects of treatment is that of premature termination. It is well established that a rather high rate of discontinuance occurs in mental health facilities. Eiduson (1968) quoted the Director of NIMH as stating that 75% of clients drop out against clinic advice after an average of 4 visits. Ross (1961), in a study of boys seen at the Pittsburgh Child Guidance Clinic, found that 28% terminated contact prematurely while Leventhal and Weinberger (1975) showed a 36.5% withdrawal rate from long-term therapy.

In the present study, case records were reviewed to determine the reasons for termination. Of the 54 treated children, 16 (30%) were withdrawn from treatment against clinic advice, 52% (28) were improved and terminated by plan, and 11% (6 cases) were terminated by the clinic because treatment was ineffective, that is, there was no evidence of progress. (Information was missing on 4 cases.)

Withdrawal from treatment has special significance in work with children. Usually children enter treatment at the instigation of adults rather than from their own sense of need or discomfort; similarly the ending of treatment and the loss of a relationship may be beyond their control. It is possible that unfinished treatment has a negative effect on the child, especially when termination occurs without his approval. If the child has formed a meaningful relationship with a therapist, the child may perceive the termination as a loss and/or rejection and an unplanned termination provides little opportunity to work through these feelings. If this were the case, the experience may add to a child's difficulties.

Kessler (1977) points out that it may be the change in a child's behavior in response to therapy that upsets parents and leads them to withdraw their child from therapy, an experience which is likely to add to the child's disturbance. Cooper and Wanerman (1977) emphasize the importance of maintaining an alliance with the family for support of the child's treatment. It is common practice to involve parents in this process in conjuction with their child's treatment for the purposes of gaining their support, enlisting them as allies in the child's therapy, modifying parent-child interaction, and reducing parental conflicts which may contribute to the child's difficulties.

Explanation of changes in the child's behavior which can be expected to grow out of treatment are an essential part of the work with parents. For example, expression of aggression, angry feelings, and conflicts are often goals of therapy with constricted children, but these changes may distress parents. If the child's new behavior leads to termination of treatment he may retreat to his former maladaptive behavior and not risk changes associated with growth.

The parents' control of the child's treatment, especially when it takes the form of ending therapy, may increase the child's sense of helplessness and lack of control, while therapy is geared to increasing his sense of competence and control. Thus, early termination may undo the positive effects of therapy and compound the child's difficulties.

In considering the effects of therapy in this research, it is important to note that only 52% of the 54 treated cases were terminated at the point improvement was recognized and a mutual plan for ending was established by clinic staff and family. In these cases therapy was terminated with adequate time to work through the ending and to consolidate gains.

In contrast, for 41% of the cases therapy was terminated by families against professional advice or by the clinic because of lack of progress. Thus, any

assessment of the effects of therapy must take into account the possible negative effects of premature termination and the potential limitation of incomplete therapy. To draw an analogy from medicine, it is clear that some illnesses that are treated by medication improve but reoccur if the prescribed
course of treatment is not completed. To assess the effects of therapy, one
must give attention to the differences between completed therapy, premature
termination, and cases terminated because child and/or family do not respond positively to the therapeutic effort. Illustrative of the latter is the work
with John H.

In the therapy process with John H. the family and Clinic invested considerable effort, but the results seemed ineffective and eventually the
parents terminated the contact.

John was referred at age 10 because of behavior problems at home and
at school, manifested in fighting with peers and siblings. His diagnosis
was severe, chronic neurotic behavior disorder, and intensive psychotherapy was undertaken. John was seen individually for 92 sessions over
a period of 1½ years. For the last 8 months he was also seen in family
therapy with his parents. Mr. and Mrs. H were seen individually and
jointly for 8 months followed by the period of family therapy.

In his therapy sessions, John attempted to get the therapist to refuse his
requests, to punish or to attack him. Therapeutic interpretations and
clarifications were percieved as attacks and often precipitated even
greater acting out and uncontrolled behavior. If the therapy sessions
were kept to superficial discussion of neutral subjects John could be
quite charming and friendly, but attempts to focus on his feelings led to
verbal or physical aggression and hostility. When the parents decided to
terminate, John indicated that he would not discuss it other than to say
he didn't want to come to therapy anyway and never had wanted to.

The parents were quite resistant when seen separately. In family sessions they came to understand that they were using John as a scapegoat.
As the parents began to alter their perceptions of John and to recognize
their own feelings, they became frightened of the need for change and
terminated treatment.

At closing, the Clinic predicted that John would have increasing difficulties of an acting out nature with possible school suspension and/or
delinquency. At follow-up John reported that he had been expelled
from high school for possession of marijuana. Conflict between John
and his parents persisted and parental threats of "kicking" him out of
the house made at the time of Clinic contact were acted on when John

was 16. John's problems became so severe that, according to his report to the interviewer, he had attempted suicide at age 20.

At follow-up John presented himself as open, honest, charming, and competent, yet there was a sociopathic quality about him. He had been moderately successful in his employment as a salesman and in this position he was his own boss, thus avoiding conflict with authority. His employment required frequent changes in location, thereby limiting his opportunity to establish relationships of much depth or long duration. John recalled his Clinic contact as something he did not like and viewed it as neither helpful nor harmful. His parents said they stopped going to the Clinic because interviews were repetitive and they weren't getting anywhere.

Characteristics of Children and Families

A second explanation for the differences in outcome between treated and untreated children might be that the children were different in significant ways before treatment began. The question then becomes: Are the different outcome ratings related to differences in the children and their families? No differences were found on a number of child and family characteristics such as diagnosis, child's severity of disturbance, age, SES, and disturbance in parents. However, the parents did differ in their response to the treatment recommendations and, according to their parents, some children in the untreated group had improved during the diagnostic evaluation or by the time treatment was available. (The average length of time between completion of diagnostic evaluation and initiation of treatment was 6.6 months with a range of 1 to 17 months.)

Clinic records were reviewed to see if reasons for differential parental response to clinic recommendations could be identified. For those children who entered treatment it is obvious that parents showed initial acceptance of the clinic's recommendation. However, the premature terminations and the fact that one third of the cases ended in less than one year suggest that even though parents initially accepted the recommendation, their participation in the process was not always maintained. When these children were treated, the early 1960s, the Clinic along with most child guidance facilities was providing long-term, open-ended treatment of about 1 to 3 years duration. Brief or planned short-term treatment was not utilized to any extent and was seldom considered in treatment recommendations. In the present study only 7 cases (25%) of planned termination occurred in less than one year, whereas 9 (60%) of the unplanned terminations occurred within one year.

In contrast, the untreated families did not enter treatment, but for several different reasons. Of considerable import, 50% of these 52 families refused treatment at the time it was recommended or offered. Twelve families gave no reason for their refusal, while 14 gave as their reason for refusal a disagreement with the clinic recommendation or a statement that the clinic had not been helpful. Several families disagreed with recommendations for hospitalization or residential treatment, while several sets of parents did not wish to be involved in treatment themselves. Five of these families accepted referrals, explored resources, but chose not to enter treatment. Even though the clinic made considerable effort to help families overcome their resistance to recommendations through outreach and additional postdiagnostic sessions, the parents continued to resist.

Jane's parents refused treatment following a period of time on the waiting list.

Jane L, a latency age child, was found to be mildly retarded with greater potential than presently evident. In addition she had a moderate to severe anxiety reaction related to several earlier traumatic events which led to fear of abandonment. The diagnostic picture was further complicated by the possibility of an endocrine disturbance. Recommendations included further medical assessment of organic factors, individual therapy for Jane, and joint treatment of parents.

In the postdiagnostic session with parents, their resistance to the recommendations was evident. In regard to the medical workup, Mrs. L expressed concern about Jane's fear of medical procedures and also about her own inability to cope with Jane's fears about medical attention. Mr. and Mrs. L expressed reluctance about involving themselves in therapy and indicated that they wished advice about coping with specific situations such as Jane's expressions of anxiety when parents went out. Mr. L stated he would have difficulty getting off work for appointments, that they could not afford the fee, and after all they just needed to use their common sense to help Jane.

The parents were offered a second appointment for further discussion of the recommendations. Mr. L did not feel this was necessary. The parents did not refuse the recommendations when given, although their reluctance was clearly evident and at the time treatment was available they declined, stating that they did not wish to involve themselves.

In contrast to this refusal group, another group of 12 families declined treatment but said they did so because they felt that the child had improved during the diagnostic study or by the time treatment was offered. Illustrative of this type of situation was an 8-year-old girl who was referred for school phobia.

Nancy T was seen at age 8 for an acute anxiety reaction manifested in a school phobia. In general Nancy appeared to be an intact child with adequate ego functions. Her anxiety stemmed from early unmet dependency needs and unresolved separation problems. Parents were concerned and were thought to be ready to involve themselves in treatment. By the time of the postdiagnostic conference Nancy had returned to school. However, parents readily acknowledged that this did not mean her problems were resolved and they expressed eagerness to enter ongoing treatment for themselves and Nancy. Treatment was offered 2 months later. At that time Mrs. T reported that Nancy was doing very well; they were not concerned about her and felt that they did not need treatment then.

At follow-up Nancy and mother remembered their contact with the Clinic. Both described a reality base for their fears, that is, the impact of being in an integrated school for the first time and Nancy's fear of a black boy who teased and threatened her. As to Clinic experience, Nancy said she saw a "middle aged man—he had dark hair—I didn't feel close to him and I couldn't tell him what was troubling me." She described the therapy room and commented: "They want you to write on the walls, but I didn't; I didn't like coming here—I was scared of it because it was different."

Despite these feelings Nancy thought the Clinic evaluation was helpful. Mrs. T felt that the diagnostic was helpful to her and helped her know how to cope with Nancy's fears, that is, Mrs. T confronted one of the youngsters who had been teasing Nancy and told him to stop.

In four instances the Clinic did not recommend therapy; one child was considered to be healthy and not in need of treatment, while three sets of parents were considered to be too disturbed to participate in the process either for themselves or in support of the child's treatment.

In summary, there were some clear differences between families who entered treatment and those who did not. These differences included attitudes toward Clinic recommendations, reactions to the diagnostic process as being helpful or unhelpful, parents' perceptions of improvements in their child, and the Clinic's assessment of a family's ability to utilize treatment.

What lies behind the varied responses of accepting and completing treatment, prematurely terminating, and refusing treatment? It is assumed that completion of treatment is related to a sense of being helped and making progress in overcoming difficulties present at the beginning of treatment. Clinic records supported this assumption in the closing notes although long-term sustainment of this progress was less evident. Also, the fact that 7 cases were closed upon Clinic recommendation because of lack of progress suggests that the treatment methods utilized were recognized as ineffective for some cases. Finally, Clinic records reflected clinical judgment of improvement or lack of it and failed to assess parents' and children's views of progress and change.

RECALL OF CLINIC EXPERIENCE

In the follow-up study an effort was made to obtain information about children's and mothers' perceptions of their Clinic experience. They were asked the open-ended question, What do you remember about going to the Clinic? This question was followed up with probes regarding why they went to the Clinic and whether or not it was helpful. Responses to these questions illuminate some important aspects of child therapy worthy of further exploration.

In general, children had minimal recall of Clinic experience. In many instances interviewers could not determine from subject reports whether the subjects had gone to the Clinic for diagnosis only or had also had treatment. However, a few subjects were specific about the service they received and others reported sufficient detail about the nature and length of the experience to determine that they had, indeed, had treatment.

Of the treated children all but four had some recall of the experience. However, only 65% were able to evaluate the helpfulness of their experience, 70% could recall something about the therapist, and 33% expressed some affect about the experience. In a comparison of treated children and those who had participated in an evaluation only, a significantly higher proportion of the treated children than the evaluation-only cases recalled their experience and considered it helpful.

The data regarding recall are suggestive rather than conclusive since there was considerable variation in the extent to which interviewers pursued information in this area and recorded it. Also, it is recognized that there is considerable variation in people's recall of events and experiences which occurred 10 to 15 years previously, especially childhood experiences. Some subjects stated that they were too young to remember or assess the effectiveness of treatment at the time it occurred. Of the 35 subjects who did respond, half considered their treatment to have been helpful and the other half thought it had not been helpful.

The subjects had some recall of the Clinic. The kinds of things they reported varied widely. Some mentioned the physical setting. They described the building as big, old, dark, and depressing and one subject recalled bars on the windows while another referred to a swing in the yard. Dislike of the one-way mirror and the idea of people being behind it and watching were reported by several subjects.

Some subjects talked about the therapist they saw. Usually they did not remember the name but did describe some physical characteristics such as sex, hair color, glasses, and so forth. Some subjects reported negative feelings about going to the Clinic. They resented going and thought it a depressing place. Difficulties about leaving school to go there were of particular concern. Several subjects stated that they had to make excuses to explain why they were leaving school and inferred that this embarrassed them.

Several subjects recalled specific aspects of their Clinic experience which was difficult for them such as being asked questions and being identified as having problems.

Lennie, age 8 at referral remembers seeing a man although he didn't remember his name. He played with clay and was asked a lot of questions. He hated the questions but thinks the experience was helpful.

Jim said he remembered "the basic ignominy and stigma of going to the clinic." He was in a boy's group and remembered the kids' and therapists' names. He stated that the therapist didn't say much and Jim and another boy did most of the talking. "I don't think the clinic was helpful but it was probably because I was bull-headed. Maybe I was too young (age 13). I tried to make my difference something special; I defended against it. I didn't open up. The doctor tried to get me to open up, but I was scared shitless. I was sure that my dad would kill me when I got home if I told about him. Dad knocked us around. He should be the one in therapy, not me. My brothers and sisters made fun of me going to a psychiatrist." Jim also said he hated the Clinic but had to go.

Don, age 13, said he disliked going to the Clinic. "I had to leave school and had to keep thinking up excuses about leaving. Also, they kept switching doctors on me." He recalled the psychological testing and repeated the first and last questions on the intelligience test. "I hated the ink blot test because I had to explain my answers. They kept asking me why I said such and such and I didn't know why. The test was too long. There were so many cards—they just kept coming at me."

How did the Clinic help these children and their parents? Some subjects indicated that the therapy experience helped them express themselves. They mentioned talking, writing, and using puppets and indicated that expression of feelings and not keeping things inside was helpful. Also, they referred to gaining an understanding of themselves, their family, and their current life situation; and they learned ways to help themselves.

Mothers found that therapy helped them to understand their children, to see them in a different light. Some mothers thought the experience led to improved communication as they learned to talk with their children. Others referred to obtaining help in relating to their children and in coping with them such as providing consistent discipline, getting off the child's back, and showing more affection. Therapy also helped some mothers to feel less guilty, to become calmer, and to be more patient than they were before therapy.

Paul was age 10 when he went to the Clinic. He and his parents had a long and successful period of therapy. Paul remembers the names but not the faces of the therapists he saw. He felt his parents learned as much as he did from the Clinic experience. Paul said he learned to talk to people. "You can't keep things inside." He said he came to the Clinic because he was "a little unstable and my parents worried about me—I constantly had trouble with people, was rebellious and nothing really interested me. I also had trouble academically." Paul concluded his comments about the Clinic with the following statement: "I learned how to help myself. I decided I was through being like I was."

Paul's mother described the Clinic experience as an unpleasant one but said it helped her, especially with the other children. "It was painful, but you can't go to the Clinic that long without picking up a few psychology tricks. I found the children needed affection. Even now, I have to premeditate upon it, but I've learned to be more affectionate and to listen to them."

In contrast to descriptions of the ways the Clinic had helped them there were also negative perceptions of the experience. In regard to the therapist they saw, some subjects stated that they didn't like him or her, that they were afraid of the therapist, they couldn't be open, didn't trust the therapist, and were afraid their parents would be told what they had said. They also expressed considerable confusion about the therapeutic process and what was expected of them such as, they didn't know what the therapist expected or what they should do there, they didn't understand the process, they hated questions, they didn't want to talk, play, or write on the walls as seemed to be expected.

These types of comments suggest that children may indeed have difficulty in understanding the therapeutic process and the respective roles of therapist and child in it. Secondly, it is possible that some therapists did not sufficiently explain and clarify the purposes and process of therapy or utilized a nondirective approach in which the main explanation was that this is the child's hour and he can do anything he wished to do in the hour.

Negative views expressed by some mothers emphasized incongruity between their expectations and what the Clinic provided. They wanted advice, specific information about the child, a prescription for ways to handle him.

Others disliked the therapist's questions which they considered intrusive, and in some instances they indicated that therapy had stirred up conflict between parents.

At the time these follow-up subjects were treated in childhood new treatment modalities of group and family treatment were being introduced; modalities which are being used extensively at present. Several subjects reported their views of these different treatment modes and their overall Clinic experience. Lack of clarity about clinic procedures and therapy are clearly evident in their reports.

Jack was not sure why his parents took him to the Clinic, perhaps because they thought some of his behavior was not normal; he got poor grades, rocked himself to sleep, and had no friends in elementary school. He went to the clinic for about three years, starting in 8th grade. Originally he saw a doctor, and then "I got shifted to another doctor and saw him for some time."

Then the family saw Mrs. Paulson for six to nine months. In individual therapy, Jack talked "but I didn't enjoy the conversation. The room we met in was for younger kids and I didn't like that. I was very much unimpressed with the whole thing." Later they started building models and he liked that. "Then they must have decided to put us all together. They must have thought they weren't making progress with me."

When they were seen in family therapy "I was able to fit into things more." He said most of the talking was done by his parents and Mrs. Paulson. Occasionally Jack would say something or Mrs. Paulson would bring him into it. He thought that was when the progress was made. "I learned about myself and family relationships."

In individual treatment Jack felt on the defensive and on guard. "The doctor asked questions to learn about me but I had no interest in learning about him." Jack felt he wasn't on the defensive in family sessions and was able to learn about himself and his family. "It eased tensions somewhat; my parents weren't as demanding on me."

Charles went to the Clinic at age 13. He disliked going and wasn't sure why his parents took him. "Maybe it was because I didn't talk to anyone." He didn't like changing therapists. "They kept switching doctors on me." First he saw a female doctor and had psychological tests. Then he saw a male, Dr. Lane. "I didn't say anything much and the doctor didn't say much either. It was an impersonal deal." The next year he was in group therapy. "That was pretty good for time passing—you could sit

there and didn't have to talk. In a group you can cover up and fake it."
Charles said he didn't know if treatment helped but he didn't like it. "To
tell the truth it didn't help; I don't know that it hurt." Charles didn't
know why treatment was started or stopped.

Both of these subjects conveyed a sense that decisions were made about treatment without their understanding them. Also, they conveyed the idea that
treatment was something done to them and not a process in which they were
actively participating. Also lacking is a conception of the therapist as a helpful, interested person or a sense of a therapeutic alliance.

Charles's mother, Mrs. A, talked at length about her Clinic experience,
including a year of family therapy. In contrast to Jack who viewed
family therapy in a positive light, Charles did not mention it. Mrs. A said
Charles was seen by psychiatrists for two years. "It didn't help at all."
Mrs. A was not seen the first year. The second year she was in group
therapy. "That was not helpful—just a bunch of women sitting around
talking."

In the third year they saw Mrs. Taylor in family sessions. Mrs. A
thought that they all gained from this. Mr. A didn't want to go, but he
did. Mrs. A learned "to control my temper, to get along with Charles
better, to see his viewpoint. We learned to understand each other—that
was helpful." Mrs. A said she also learned to understand why she did
things and what she should or shouldn't do. Mrs. A added, "Mrs. Taylor
seemed more interested in us while the others treated us like doctor-
patient; that is, they were cold and treated us almost like objects."

In summary, the recall data suggest confusion about the therapeutic process,
reflected in terms of either not understanding or knowing what to expect or
what was expected of them or having expectations that were not met by the
experience. Comments focused on the respective roles and responsibilities of
therapist and patient. The relationship between patients' perceptions of
psychotherapy and outcome is an area for further research attention.

Research concerning adults' perceptions of therapeutic experiences has
focused on their judgments of the helpfulness of therapy and therapist characteristics. Work on children's views of therapeutic experiences is minimal.
Levy's (1969) follow-up study of formerly hospitalized children refers to some
global impressions of the total experience. Koch (1973) did a survey of analysts and asked them for reports of contacts with former child analytic patients. The analysts reported on contacts with 22 former patients. The patients
were seen most often within one year of termination, but the time of their con-

tact varied from one to sixteen years. Most viewed the analyst as a real person, a grown-up friend who was kindly, interested, and understanding. Specific aspects of the analytic work tended to be repressed.

Meyer (1975) held follow-up interviews with 25 adolescents who had been seen for an average of 10.7 sessions. Follow-up occurred from two weeks to three months after termination. About half (13) of these adolescents thought therapy had been helpful, 9 indicated ambivalence, and 3 stated it was not helpful. The adolescents' comments about the therapeutic experience focused on their relationship with and perception of the therapist. Those who viewed therapy as helpful reported liking the therapist, being comfortable or relaxed in the relationship, sensing the therapist as a real, caring human being. They felt understood by their therapists, felt they could trust them, and were close to them, yet felt autonomous in what was seen as a two-way relationship. Some referred to the youthfulness of their therapists as a positive attribute which contributed to their being understood. In contrast, those who were ambivalent felt that the therapist didn't care, that the human element was lacking, and that the relationship was distant and not comforting or supportive.

The importance of a meaningful relationship characterized by warmth, caring, and understanding were clearly evident in these studies as well as the present research. The extent to which such a relationship is achieved may be influenced by the nature of the child's difficulties, his capacity to relate, and the therapist's personality and skill in conveying the purpose of the therapeutic process and in setting the stage for ongoing work together.

SELECTION OF CASES FOR TREATMENT

What are the criteria for selecting children and their families for treatment? Is the fact that a family is referred to a clinic and goes through an evaluation process sufficient reason to recommend that they be treated? Clinic practice seemed to be predicated on the assumption that most referred children were moderately to severely disturbed and in need of treatment.

This assumption of disturbance and a need for treatment overlooks several important factors. First, the evaluation process itself may have sufficient therapeutic effects to free the child for further growth and to enable parents to support their child's growth and to help him overcome difficulties. Secondly, some parents are unable to involve themselves in therapy or to provide support to the child's therapy. Third, the degree of health or the transitory nature of symptoms may be obscured by the pathological orientation of clinics. Finally, the discrepant views and expectations of therapy held by children, parents, and mental health professionals may interfere with the establishment of working alliances essential to effective treatment.

In this study families participated in an extensive evaluation process which consisted of at least three interviews with parents, three interviews with the child, two psychological testing sessions, and one or more postdiagnostic interviews. In this process family members examined their interaction with each other, their expectations regarding each person's functioning, and feelings and attitudes toward themselves and others. Not infrequently parents acquired increased understanding of their children and tried out different ways of relating to them. Direct suggestion and advice were sometimes offered.

The fact that 12 families reported improvement in their children during or after the evaluation supports the possibility that the evaluation process in itself was helpful to the child and his parents. On the other side, 14 families disagreed with the diagnostic recommendations and/or considered the Clinic to be unhelpful, and for 22 families no information about their reasons for not entering treatment was available.

The following case is illustrative of the therapeutic effects of the evaluations.

Steve was referred to the Clinic by the school because of underachievement. His grades fluctuated considerably, an indication that he had good potential but that anxiety was interfering with learning. Testing showed considerable anxiety and phobic elements along with concerns about sexual identity. Parents had a stable marriage of 20 years duration and were concerned, conscientious people. All members of the family were frightened of feelings, especially those of hostility and aggression.

Steve reflected the family pattern by being a "too good," sweet, 9-year-old boy. His diagnosis was neurotic reaction.

At postdiagnostic interview the parents expressed pleasure with Steve's improvement, especially his report card. The parents felt this change was related to the evaluation. They said Steve had been pleased about coming to the Clinic and expressed enthusiasm as he went through the process. They said he liked the doctor very much. Both parents reported that they were trying to stop their overprotection of Steve. They were giving him more freedom to come and go such as letting him ride his bicycle more places, letting him go to Saturday afternoon movies, and encouraging him to go out with other children. Mrs. J said she had become aware of how close she and Steve had been and she was trying to loosen this tie.

In general, the parents were cooperative and nondefensive. They could see their overprotectiveness and moved quickly to lessen this. They seemed eager to enter treatment and accepted assignment to the waiting list. They chose not to enter treatment when it was offered. At follow-up Steve was rated as well functioning. He remembered the doctor he had seen at the Clinic and both Steve and Mrs. J thought the Clinic experience had been helpful.

It is evident that not all parents are willing or able to participate in therapy on behalf of their children. However, clinicians seem to be persistent in trying to involve parents and to engage them in ongoing work, even though the parents might resist and eventually terminate prematurely, a sequence which might have negative effects on the child. In the present study only 3 cases were considered untreatable because of parental limitations or resistance. However, Clinic records clearly indicated that other parents might be unable to utilize clinic services and the number of premature terminations supported this assessment. The factor of a mother's recognition of her role in her child's pathology was significantly related to outcome in Lessing's (1966) study.

The discrepancy between client expectations and the nature of clinical service is closely related to the issue of parents' treatability. For instance, it is not uncommon for parents to deliver their children to a clinic to be "fixed" or changed and often they expect this to occur rather quickly. In contrast, mental health professionals are likely to view the children's problems as growing out of difficulties in the parent-child interaction, reactive to stress in the parents' lives or indicative of a displacement of individual parent personality problems or of marital conflict. Consequently, services often focus on parents as individuals, on the marital relationship, and on their feelings, attitudes, and behavior toward their children. This shift in focus from parental concerns, anxiety, and sometimes anger about their children to their own behavior, feelings, and attitudes may be both confusing and threatening to parents.

For children, the therapeutic process is clearly foreign to them; it is outside the realm of any previous experience. Consequently, they are confronted with an unknown situation which may be colored by fantasies and by their parents' explanation of the service. Under the best of circumstances, the child associates going to a clinic with some unacceptable behavior on his part and in some instances clinic service has been presented to him as a threat and a punishment. The clinic contact singles out the child as different from his siblings or peers, a feeling not enjoyed by children of most ages. Thus, clinicians have a major task in making the therapeutic process understandable to the child so that he can participate constructively in it. Clarification of his expectations and those of the therapist becomes essential.

Finally, clinicians tend to weight the therapeutic hour as all-important in the life of the child. Alternatives to therapy to enhance the child's growth may be considered, but are usually viewed as supplemental to the therapy. Included among these alternatives are special school placements, after-school activities, and growth-producing contacts with other adults such as teachers and relatives. For instance, Heinicke and Goldman (1960) draw attention to the possibility that a series of life experiences or therapeutic contact can lead to more adequate adjustment.

The high percentage of children judged to be in need of treatment, all but one in this study, suggests that a child is considered disturbed merely by virtue of being referred to a clinic. This idea overlooks the possibility of clinics providing preventive service. Popular literature and the movement toward parent education suggest that parents give attention to their parental role in facilitating their child's growth. Clinics could provide a useful consultation service to families to determine whether a child's behavior is indicative of a transitory developmental phase or is evidence of structured pathology. Clinic staffs, with their emphasis on fantasy and unconscious conflicts, may overlook the child's ego capacities and adaptive traits and recommend unneeded treatment. Again, the long tradition of a disease orientation may obscure the relative balance of healthy and unhealthy forces in the child's personality and in his life situation.

In summary, other research as well as this study on child therapy outcome suffers from serious methodological problems. These problems are well identified by Heinicke and Strassman (1975). Nevertheless, evidence is available to support the idea that most child disorders remit without treatment (Rutter, 1975). Moreover, the goals of therapy cannot be measured by global assessments of outcome, nor do most measures of this kind take into account the important role of therapy pointed out by Rutter (1975), that is, to relieve current suffering and to hasten recovery. Although long-term results of treated and untreated children may be similar, the duration and suffering associated with childhood difficulties are certainly worthy of clinical intervention.

Most research has focused on treatment results with quite heterogeneous populations. The need for controlled studies of treatment with specific types of difficulties and diagnoses as well as with specific age groups is clearly indicated. The goals of therapy for each child need to be established and outcome related to them. Further, the impressions derived from review of case records and subjects' recall of therapy experience suggests a need for more attention to be given in work with children to exploring and clarifying the therapeutic process. Results are likely to be best when the child is an active participant in the process and when he and the therapist have established goals for their work together.

The possibility that the extent of the therapist's experience is related to results, as was evident in this research, suggests the need for further exploration of this variable. If experience is a significant factor, what can be done in training to help overcome the experience limitation? Perhaps beginning therapists need a period of time in which to prepare themselves for therapeutic work with children before undertaking it. This preparation might include role-playing, observing experienced therapists at work, especially on videotape, and talking directly with children of various ages outside a clinic setting.

Finally, a number of interrelated treatment variables may be related in combination but not individually to outcome. Research is needed in which there is adequate control of these variables and/or in which their relative weight can be assessed. These variables include: therapist's experience, number of therapists, length of therapy, and planned or premature termination. In addition, outcome measures are needed which take into consideration the Strupp and Hadley (1977) tripartite model of mental health which includes societal, patient, and mental health perspectives.

CHAPTER 8

Implications And Recommendations for Mental Health Services for Children

There is now a growing interest in providing adequate mental health service for children. The pressure on government and private agencies to recognize and respond to the needs of children comes from a society which is becoming increasingly aware of the cost to itself of mental illness, from the mental health professionals who believe that their services may decrease the incidence of mental illness and social maladjustment in the adult population, and from the planners who seek the most efficient and economical ways to improve services and provide new ones. The need for services is well documented. The question still to be resolved is what kinds of children should be served and what types of services would be best suited to meet the needs that society is beginning to recognize and express?

Answers to this question have been sought through this and other research and while there is, now, a growing body of knowledge to guide the mental health effort, there remain many areas for which no answers have been found. Sometimes the researcher is stymied by a lack of available methodology to handle statistically the complexity of variables that must be considered; sometimes he is confounded by variables outside his control. But more often his frustration is likely to arise from the lack of predictability in the human organism itself and in its milieu. Children, unlike hothouse plants, move and vary their environments, produce as well as respond to changes in others, and more often surprise those who predict their future rather than confirm their hypotheses.

Although clinicians are often accused of lagging behind the researchers in changing their services to correspond to latest research findings, the extent to which such changes are warranted is limited by the ambiguity of the findings and by the lack of faith in alternate modes of dealing with clinical problems. Even research such as this which has been carefully planned and executed comes up with relationships such as those between childhood characteristics and adult outcome which are only modestly significant and minimally predictive. Moreover, they are based on probability statistics of groups whereas the clinician is faced with the responsibility of recommendations for each child who comes into his office.

This probability for success in the clinical situation has been compared to that in the industrial situation (Meehl, 1954). The industrial employer simply bases his selection and promotion practice on his best chances for success as understood from prior experience in that industry under similar circumstances. He worries little or not at all about the applicants or employees who are eliminated by the "chance-for-success" formulae. The clinician, on the other hand, must seriously concern himself about every child and cannot avoid wondering if, perhaps, the child whom he might eliminate from service on the basis of research probability for success might indeed be the one, like many of the examples in this book, who defies the prediction made for him through group statistics.

One criterion of need for service is, of course, the probability of maladjustment in adulthood. Another less emphasized but equally important criterion involves the child's present discomfort and/or suffering; the extent to which his symptoms and behavior are disrupting his functioning in his family, school, and community; and the degree to which growth and personality development have been blocked or regression has occurred.

The proponents of clinical services for children see these services as a means of preventing maladjustment and mental illness in adulthood. The assumptions that there *is* continuity of disturbance from childhood to adulthood and that early detection and intervention can interrupt this continuity have been the stimuli for this and other follow-up research as well as the basis for children's clinical services. These assumptions have only recently been challenged.

Several researchers (Kohlberg et al., 1972), impressed by findings on the lack of continuity into adulthood of many childhood disturbances and by the seeming ineffectiveness of child psychotherapy, would advise an alternate solution to the "heavy concentration of these services on a few children through diagnosis and treatment" (p. 1273). The alternate solution proposed by Kohlberg and his colleagues is a more community mental health or reeducation approach to mental health services, wherein an environment can be created "in which the coping and ego development of all children are facilitated. . ." (p. 1273). These authors also suggest, however, that children with problems should receive more attention than those without manifest problems and children with severe problems should receive more than those with less severe problems. They do not suggest that this "attention" should necessarily be psychotherapy; on the contrary, they propose that psychotherapy requires more ego maturity than most children possess and should be delayed.

While agreeing, in principle, that research findings cast grave doubts on the continuity of most disturbances into adulthood and on the efficacy of traditional outpatient services for children as they are now operated, the results of the research reported in this book do not warrant the rejection of these services. In the first place, the clinics may provide immediate relief to children and, more especially, to parents, even if the results are not crucial to adult adjustment. The problems of childhood need not be permanent to warrant interventive effort. As Robins (1972) points out, "no one would think of evaluating the effectiveness of medical treatment by seeing how many attenders of a general medical clinic are well or improved a year or two later while comparing them with people who approached the clinic for treatment but were not seen" (p. 428). She points out that for many self-limited illnesses, such as influenza, from which *all* patients will have recovered, the relevant question is whether "the course of the disease was milder as a result of treatment" (p. 428). In addition, it is likely that reductions in symptoms and disturbed behavior will enhance the child's opportunity to find environmental supports, especially in the form of interpersonal relationships, that will promote his growth toward maturity.

Secondly, and more importantly, while the efficacy of clinical services is not proven, neither is that of other approaches. The reports of at least two school-based projects (Gildea et al., 1967; Cowen et al., 1973) do not show positive results with less intensive and less expensive approaches.

SELECTION OF CHILDREN FOR CLINIC SERVICE

It is evident from the body of research now available that many children who reach child guidance are not as seriously disturbed as they are judged to be by societal agents and clinic personnel and certainly not so disturbed as to warrant the long and expensive course of treatment that is too often recommended. Yet this and other research attest to the fact that a substantial proportion of the children who reach the Clinics are indeed headed for maladjustment in adulthood and that the proportion is much higher than that in the general population. In this research, 92, or 46%, of the 200 children evaluated and followed up were moderately to severely maladjusted in adulthood and most of them had been so identified in the clinic conference. They needed *some* kind of help and the only question is whether or not they received what they needed. Moreover, it has been estimated, from school surveys, that for every child referred to clinics five equally disturbed children never see a clinic. When these two findings are combined with that of the stage-specific nature of many childhood problems, it becomes clear that the clinics must select their clientele more carefully to assure that those who get this specialized kind of service are really in need of it, and, thus, to make room for the many children to whom service is not now available.

This discriminating selection requires better screening at the referral stage. The literature, including this report, offers guidelines for better screening, including, for example, more service for antisocial children in the initial stages of acting out behavior and the identification of children with other serious problems early in life. One large group of neglected children are lower class, underprivileged children whose family and educational settings do not provide awareness of and resources for their mental health needs. Middle class children—especially those with neurotic symptomatology—are probably too often referred to clinics when, as shown in research, most of them grow into healthy adults even without special help.

Implications for Procedures Within Clinic Service

These research results agree with those of many other recent studies to point to an urgent need for better diagnostic evaluation and more selective recommendations within child guidance. Ernest Kris and Anna Freud insisted that accurate assessment in childhood is the first requirement for prediction and, thus, for useful recommendation. They both point up, however, the extreme difficulty in achieving accurate assessment and diagnosis and various additional obstacles such as the unpredictability of environmental happenings, changes in the rate of maturational progress (after diagnostic assessment), and the self-healing qualities of further development. Their pessimism about prediction has found support in follow-up results. Even with the detailed diagnostic material available to the authors, few clearcut guidelines to prediction can be formulated.

Foremost among the implications from the research is that a professional team in conference does a better job in diagnosing and judging severity of childhood disturbance than psychologists or psychiatrists, rating from clinical material, do separately. The conference rating of intensity of disturbance significantly differentiated those children who remained disturbed from those who were (and remained) relatively healthy and it also differentiated those who went from less to greater disturbance from those who improved in adulthood. This superiority may be, at least in part, due to the contribution of the social worker at the conference and the consideration of factual information from parents and schools. The research social worker was able, from recorded social history, school reports, application data, and symptom lists, to arrive at a rating of social adjustment which proved to be the best predictor of social adjustment at follow-up.

The findings point to a need to combine clinical diagnosis with other variables such as severity of disturbance, age, sex, and intellectual assets. The findings also suggest that the psychiatrist and especially the psychologist may put too much faith in fantasy material in diagnostic formulation, at least in terms of the usefulness of the formulation for prediction to later adjustment. From a clinical point of view, it may be that psychological testing could be better used for treatment purposes in those cases where the therapist needs a clear understanding of the internal dynamics of the child than for diagnosis and prediction. The use of the clinical, dynamic formulation for predictive purposes is by no means, of course, the intent of most service settings and many professionals with a psychodynamic orientation profess *not* to have social adjustment as their goal in making recommendations. The discussion in this text of Strupp and Hadley's tripartite model (1977) is germane to this difference in goals.

Related to the importance of social and behavioral data for predictive purposes is a suggestion that more attention should be given in the assessment to school reports and even to actual observation of the child in the school setting as he interacts with peers. The finding that several school behaviors are related to outcome, especially antisocial behaviors, has implication also for helping teachers in consultation and in making appropriate referrals.

Teachers are somewhat better informants than parents when outcome is the criterion. Parents tended to be critical of their children, citing many more symptoms than did teachers and, in general, painting a gloomy picture of their feelings about this particular child and about their marital relationships. These findings lead to the suggestion that clinicians may be too impressed by parental reports of specific behaviors and, especially, that it is necessary to sift out stage-specific behaviors, that is, behaviors normal for that stage, even though they are bothersome to the parent, from those behaviors that are not normal for the stage and those that have persisted for a long time without abatement.

Clinicians also need to be aware that the latency age period (about 7 through 10), which *is* unfortunately the most frequent age for clinic referral, is not a period from which prediction is accurately made. It is probably not by chance, however, that most referrals are made at this age period. Children, particularly boys, at this age, present problems at school and at home which are especially bothersome to adults. On the other hand, few children of age 4 to 6 years are referred to clinics and yet there was, in this research, a definite relationship between poor outcome in adulthood and parents' *noticing* problems in the earliest years.

In almost all outpatient settings, moreover, the ratio of boys to girls is high and yet this ratio does not hold up in adulthood. Research results suggest that the kinds of problems which relate, in girls, to serious maladjustment in later life do not, in general, get them to clinics in childhood.

That many childhood problems are age-specific cannot be stressed sufficiently. Along with the finding that problems predictive of poor outcome in boys are, for the most part, different from those in girls, age-relatedness has implications not only for clinic practice but also for parent and teacher education. For clinic practice, it points to the possibility that parents might be helped, early in the diagnostic process, to become aware of what to expect in behavior at each stage of development and to handle "normal" behaviors better. In this connection, one wonders if many of the parents who terminated clinic service without therapy *did*, in fact, gain these insights from the diagnostic process and even, to some degree, from filling out the lengthy application and symptom-behavior forms. If this is true, it might help to account for the relatively good outcome of nontreated children in the sample.

The Child Guidance Clinic from which this research originated, like many other medically based clinics, was oriented toward assessing pathology, and when the research forms were initiated, little attention was paid to assessing strengths. This deficit has undoubtedly limited the conclusions that can be drawn from the results, especially in regard to the possibility that many of the children who did not deteriorate or who improved in spite of severe problems may have done so because of (unassessed) strengths in personality structure and/or functioning. The few assets which were assessed, such as IQ, did correlate in some measure with outcome. (The correlation was reduced by the exclusion from the sample of children with IQs below 75.) The importance of cognitive assets to good outcome is well documented in the research literature (Havighurst, 1962; Kohlberg, 1972). It is likely that if these and other assets (for example, efficiency of defenses, resiliency, intactness of family) were given more weight in clinical assessment that less dire predictions for the majority of children and less frequent recommendations for long-term, intensive therapy would be made.

IMPROVEMENT OF SERVICES TO CHILDREN

If the results of this research and several other studies which addressed themselves to the effectiveness of therapy could be taken at face value, the implications might be that psychotherapy is not warranted for children in outpatient clinics. About two thirds of such samples are found to improve with or without psychotherapy. Actually, however, adequate research designed to contrast a treated group with a truly comparable control group and to regulate therapist and therapy variables has not yet been done. Moreover, it is impossible to evaluate in any meaningful way the results of therapy for those children for whom it should not have been recommended in the first place. Again, the inadequacy of diagnostic assessment must be recognized.

In the sample of this research, practically *all* (97%) of the children evaluated at the Clinic were recommended for therapy. Thus, *no* differential selection was employed and it is not known how many of the children who did *not* need therapy were in the group who received it and how many such children were in the group who did not. If the negative findings on therapy outcome, undependable as they are, have any applicability, it must be that recommendations of all kinds should be considered to suit the many levels of disturbance, the different assets and liabilities of the children and their families, the probability of success with different syndromes, the capacity for utilization of therapy in both the child and his parents, and the growth potential of children. Although some clinics make an honest effort to assess these factors, too often the final recommendation still turns out to be psychotherapy, usually of the child individually.

That some children benefit from therapy is evident in immediate and long-term effects, shown in individual cases reported in this and other research and in those cases described by clinicians from their own practice experience. However, the effectiveness of individual treatment might be enhanced not only by improved selectivity of children for treatment but by additional emphasis on certain aspects of the therapeutic process.

First, the subjective descriptions of children's recall of therapeutic experiences point to confusion about the process and to negative feelings about being singled out as needing mental health services. Several approaches to these problems are warranted. Within the therapeutic process there is need for repeated clarification with the child of the reasons why he is participating in therapy, the purposes and goals of the therapeutic work, and the mutual responsibilities and expectations of child and therapist in their contacts with each other. Furthermore, there is need to address, at both a societal level and in the ongoing therapeutic work with individual children, the negative attitudes associated with utilization of mental health services. Obviously, continuing public education regarding mental health problems and services is indicated through mass media and through special projects carried out within public school systems in order to reach all children. In addition, mental health information and education services should be provided for parents, teachers, and other adults who are in frequent and meaningful contact with children.

For example, Blatt and Starr (1977) reported a project in which a community guidance center and a public school which contained a sizeable high risk population cooperated in providing outreach mental health services. Clinic staff assigned to the school provided consulation to teachers, assessments of children, and individual, group, and family therapy to clients in their own homes and in the school setting. They reached families who usually were unwilling to follow through on referrals to the regular clinic setting.

A somewhat different approach was utilized by McGarrity (1975) in an effort to minimize children's negative attitudes toward counseling services by developing avenues for social worker-child relationships to start before problems evolved. He met with students in classroom groups for sessions focused on feelings, that is, the importance of feelings and the need to share and understand them. Through discussion, role play, and drawing activities with the students, they became acquainted with the social worker, accepted him as a caring person, and began to use him to discuss immediate problems and concerns.

The child in therapy might be helped through exploration of his fantasies and fears about "being sick" or "being different," through repeated clarification of his distorted perception of mental health problems, and through support to him in finding ways to cope with questions and comments from peers and adults in regard to his involvement in therapy.

A second area for major attention is that of actually engaging those in need of treatment in the process and in maintaining their participation to its completion. Certainly such engagement and completion would be facilitated by the information, education, and clarification recommended above. In addition, there is a need for full assessment of parents' ability to support their child's treatment and to cooperate in it and for establishment of parental commitment to completion of treatment. These are not easy tasks when so often the parents of troubled children are themselves faced with overwhelming problems, external stress, and limited resources. What is called for is the use of clinical expertise or authority along with a strong supportive relationship and cognitive explanation of anticipated immediate and long-term effects of therapy.

If, as theory seems to indicate, it is important that treatment be carried to completion, then it is logical to evaluate carefully the length of time a particular child and his family need to participate in it to obtain meaningful changes. In general, clinics are oriented to providing long-term and open-ended treatment and short-term, limited treatment. Several projects on short-term treatment show results comparable to longer term intervention. Little attention is given to treatment of duration between these two extremes.

Until clinicians, families, and society can achieve some consensus on the goals of treatment and identify criteria for assessing the achievement of such goals, services will continue to be carried on needlessly or without clarity as to their effectiveness or completion. Further development and use of the Strupp and Hadley (1977) tripartite model of mental health should provide guidelines for assessing achievement of therapeutic goals.

Alternatives to Individual Therapy. Clinic services to children have gradually expanded during recent years to include prevention and early detection through educational and consultative services to such groups as parents, teachers, and child care workers. In addition, there are out-reach services designed to work with high risk populations. The extent and variety of such services are limited; research methodology to assess the effects of preventive programs is still in an early development phase. Nevertheless, it is essential to continue to formulate and assess various approaches to prevention, to early detection and treatment of children's problems, and to the promotion of normal growth and development.

In addition to these broader programs, several recommendations are made for alternatives to individual, family, or group treatment of those children who actually reach child guidance clinics for evaluation and possible treatment.

The diagnostic process could be considered a consultation service to parents in which the focus would be on identifying the resources within the child, his family, school, and community that might be enlisted to promote his developmental processes and to overcome current problems. This could be done through providing parents and/or teachers with the following: 1) exploring the meaning and purposes a child's behavior serves; 2) describing the kinds of relationships and experiences a particular child needs; and 3) giving direct advice and suggesting actions that significant persons in the child's life might take to be of help to him.

Thus, major focus of diagnosis would be on determining ways in which a child's problems and needs could be handled within his current or potential network of relationships. This approach does not exclude therapy as a possible diagnostic recommendation, but suggests that other ways of helping a child in addition to or separate from psychotherapy be consistently considered as part of routine clinic procedures. Such is not the practice in many clinics and the specific suggestion here is toward a reorientation of clinical staff from the primacy of direct treatment to an emphasis on selective use of a wide range of interventive approaches.

What seems necessary, in the present state of our knowledge, is that a *network* of various kinds of facilities and services be developed so that children with various levels and extent of needs can be served appropriately. Such a plan is clearly outlined in the 1972 report of the Joint Information Service, *Children and Mental Health Centers* (Glasscote et al). After a national survey of government supported services for children, the JIS survey team saw the need for many different approaches to caring for mental health needs from general resource building through better environmental and educational programs for children through parent-training and guidance to intensive psychotherapy and even residential treatment for children who are already showing signs of serious illness. With such a full network of services available, the place of the child guidance clinic would not be the catchall that it now represents but, rather, its more specific functions could be defined and more time would be available for children who do need its services.

Continued postdiagnostic work with parents and periodic follow-up of children are also recommended as alternatives to child therapy. Focus of parental guidance should be to develop an understanding of their child's behavior, especially its possible stage-specific nature, and in some cases, toward acceptance of his individuality. This service to parents should be accompanied by regular, periodic contact with the child to be sure that the problems were indeed stage-specific or transitory and have diminished rather than escalated over time. Such monitoring of children's development would provide opportunity for relevant intervention, if necessary, and would free staff time for treatment of families and children with more severe or entrenched problems.

RESEARCH IMPLICATIONS

The major thrust of this research was on prediction, while secondary emphasis was placed on therapy outcome. The complexity of these two processes, as well as the methodological issues inherent in designing research to resolve them, are well stated by review articles written by Kohlberg et al. (1972), Robins (1972), and Heinicke and Strassman (1975). Nevertheless, cumulative evidence is emerging to suggest further research efforts.

It is time to bring together the findings of follow-back, longitudinal, and prospective studies and to make use of these findings in routine clinic practice to provide a data base for future research. Factors such as social functioning (especially peer relationships), clinical diagnosis, severity of disturbance, and degree and type of anxiety have potential predictive value. However, there must be other factors not yet identified which contribute to diverse outcomes for children with the same characteristics and diagnoses.

Of particular importance is the need to design studies that control sex and age variables since certain behaviors or characteristics have opposite effects for boys and girls and some evidence indicates that specific behaviors at one age may be related to adult maladjustment whereas the same behaviors at other ages may be associated with future health.

Of particular note is the need for research on latency age children, the period when the majority of children are referred for clinic services but the age-period least predictive to later adjustment. One promising lead for such research is the finding that some outcome patterns are predictable on the basis of reversals of characteristics between two successive age periods (e.g., Peskin, 1972). Thus, latency age characteristics may be important to outcome mainly in relation to development in succeeding stages.

There is a need to identify syndromes of childhood disturbance which are important; yet the failure of statistical procedures, especially group statistics, to predict specific outcomes is recognized. Predictions of adult outcome, for each child seen in mental health clinics, based on a synthesis of data derived from varied sources and including clinical judgments should be included in objective form in all clinic records to provide a basis for discovering which variables do and which do not contribute to prediction.

Finally, therapy outcome studies must be designed to control therapy variables such as type of treatment, duration, experience of therapist, reason for termination, and child variables such as age, sex, symptoms, and clinical diagnosis. Research on therapy needs to include, moreover, an assessment of parents' involvement in and response to treatment as well as that of their children. The researcher should plan purposefully and report clearly the time at which effects of therapy are assessed, such as at the point of termination or 5 to 10 years later; and the criteria for outcome should be definitely stated, for example, in terms of improvement versus absolute level of adjustment.

Although child guidance clinics have, in the past, emphasized the need for an intensive and comprehensive diagnostic process as the basis for planning remedial service and especially for psychotherapy, deliberate use of specific diagnostic findings to guide interventive efforts seems often to have been neglected. In the Clinic where this research originated, for example, recommendations for psychotherapy resulted almost indiscriminately from the diagnostic studies; the psychological and/or psychiatric results seem not to have been used regularly by therapists. While the variables from psychological testing and psychiatric interviewing chosen for this project seem to have little predictive value as far as *outcome* is concerned, it is conceivable that they may contribute much to the understanding of the child's "inner" dynamic life, an understanding which is usually considered necessary for successful analytically oriented therapy.

Unfortunately, the Clinic records did not include data on each case as to whether or not the diagnostic formulations were used in the course of therapy, and this variable could not be included in the study of therapy outcome. This variable might be included in research designed to assess the success of therapy. It may be that a lack of understanding of the child's dynamics, especially by trainees who have limited experience, is one contributor to the failure to demonstrate effectiveness of psychotherapy.

So far, these recommendations have centered on ways to increase clinic efficiency by screening out those who, it seems from research findings, can do without or with *less* expensive services and still attain an acceptable adult adjustment; and on alternatives to long-term individual therapy. There is, unfortunately, much research evidence that, as yet, no procedures, therapy or others, have proven effective for that group of outpatient referrals with psychosis and *severe* antisocial behaviors who make up the bulk of the one third who do *not* recover. The implications for these groups are for *earlier* recognition and for persistent, formalized, experimental and programmatic research to find ways of intervening to disrupt the continuity of their disorders. These are the children, after all, who will grow up and force society to recognize their needs.

Clinic Forms For Childhood Data

Three of the forms utilized for obtaining data at the original clinic evaluation, as well as the definitions of diagnostic categories utilized, are included here. Only the major items contained in the forms without the precoded categories are presented; the full forms with the codes are available from the authors.

APPLICATION FORM

1. Name
2. Address
3. Date of application
4. Child's age
5. Child's birthdate
6. Sex
7. Grade
8. Do you live in St. Louis City or County?
9. Name of person who suggested referral
10. What is main reason for bringing child to clinic?
11. What do you feel child's difficulties are? (*Describe in detail.*)
12. Information for male and female head of household:
    Name
    Age and birthdate
    Education
    Occupation
    Place of employment
    Yearly income
13. Children in family:
    Name
    Age
    Sex

Birthdate

Grade

14. Others living in household:
Name
Sex
Age
Education
Relationship to Patient

15. Does either parent have children by another marriage?

16. Age of child when you first noticed the problem

17. Who first noticed the problem?

18. Who first suggested you seek help for the child?

19. Who suggested you come to the clinic at this time?

20. Child's race

21. Relationship to child of person filling out application

22. Birth order of child

23. Child is single birth or twin?

24. Child is being raised by?

25. If child is adopted indicate:
Age of adoption
Age came into your home
Source child obtained from

26. Marital status of natural parents

27. Religious background of mother, father

28. Religious faith in which child is being raised

29. Type of present residence

30. Number or previous residences since child's birth

31. Number of people living in present household

32. Number of adults (over age 16) and children (age 16 or under) living in present household

33. Years grandparents have lived in family since child's birth

34. Hometown of male and female heads of household

35. Number of hours worked per week—male and female heads of household

DEVELOPMENTAL QUESTIONNAIRE

1. Mother's physical condition during pregnancy.

2. Mother's emotional reaction to pregnancy.

3. Bleeding during pregnancy.

4. Infectious diseases during pregnancy.

5. Was child a full-term newborn?

6. Was child placed in an incubator?

7. Was labor natural, induced, caesarian?

8. Were instruments used because of difficult labor?

9. Duration of labor.

10. Type of anesthesia or medication for child's birth.

11. What part of child was born first?

12. Birth weight.

13. Condition of baby immediately after birth.

14. How was child fed?

15. If breast fed, were there any difficulties?

16. If bottle fed, were there any formula problems?

17. Baby's response to feeding.

18. Did the baby have spells of colic?

19. Did the baby have spells of constipation?

20. Did the baby have spells of diarrhea?

21. What attitude or mood did the baby seem to express most of the time? For example: happy; smiling and laughing; "cuddly"; clinging; whiney; seemed in pain; sad. Please describe in more detail.

22. During the first year how active was child?

23. During the first year was there anything (even if it had nothing to do with baby) that caused unhappiness or anxiety or placed mother or father under specific strain?

24. Did child ever show any of the following behavior consistently over a period of time? (Banged head, rocked, pulled hair out, bit self, etc.)

25. Did child have angry outbursts, temper tantrums, or similar kinds of behavior which caused you concern? (*Describe.*)

26. Was either parent out of the home for a period longer than six months? (After child was born to 6 years of age)

27. Did child ever lose any person through death with whom he (she) seemed to have a close relationship?

28. If child did lose any person through death, indicate age of child when this occurred. (*List for each person.*)

29. List illnesses child has had. State age at which each occurred, how long each illness lasted, what treatment was given, and if there were any unusual reactions or after-effects.

30. Did child have any operations such as: circumcision, tonsillectomy, adenoidectomy?

31. What accidents did child have?

32. Is child on any medication now?

SYMPTOM LIST

DIRECTIONS: Read each statement below and underline all the sentences or phrases that describe yourself _____ ; your son _____ , or daughter _____ .

NO.

1. 1. Occasionally wakens at night; awakens early, or has difficulty in going to sleep.

2. Occasional nightmares; periodically awakens, afraid; periodically wanders about the house during the night; excessive talking during sleep; restless sleep; wets in sleep; wakes up tired and often cross; tends to sleep more than normal.

3. Frequent night terrors; lies awake hours before falling asleep; spends much time sleeping; always tired.

4. Because of the problems above he (she) frequently stays up all night; has night terrors; loss of sleep to the extent health is impaired; sedatives are frequently required.

5. Other (specify) _____

2. 1. Has a few food dislikes, but generally eats well; occasionally skips meals or overeats.

2. Has many dislikes or preferences; does not generally eat well; goes for a day or two at a time without a regular meal.

3. Has numerous food fads or keeps away from certain foods (milk, eggs, etc.); for long periods eats only a few foods; eats very little or excessively; goes for weeks at a time eating practically nothing; stomach frequently upset; frequent and intense vomiting; markedly over- or underweight; so serious as to require a physician's advice.

4. Can't keep anything down; vomits to degree hospitalization is required; has to be tube fed or fed through veins; problem of eating to the extent that health is impaired.

5. Other (specify) _____

3. 1. Mouths objects before going to sleep or occasionally when engaged in interesting activity.

2. Sometimes mouths objects when quiet or inactive or with family or friends.

3. Sucks thumb or mouths objects usually at all times and all places

when not otherwise engaged; mouths objects to the extent that mouth is sore and requires treatment.

4. Is so involved with mouthing objects that it severely limits opportunity for social activities and relationships.

5. Other (specify) _____

4.   1. After normal training age is dry during the day but wets occasionally at night.

2. Wets occasionally during the day; wets frequently at night.

3. Wets often during the day; wets almost every night.

4. Wetting keeps the child from being with friends or going to camp.

5. Other (specify) _____

5.   1. After normal training age occasionally soils during the day or night under specific stress or illnesses; goes a day or two without a bowel movement.

2. Occasionally soils (weekly); sometimes withholds bowel movements for as long as a week.

3. Withholds all bowel movements for as long as a week; frequently soils; never, or almost never, has movements in toilet.

4. Needs to be hospitalized or frequently needs physician's attention because of his bowel control problem.

5. Other (specify) _____

6.   1. In school, is not achieving to capacity in one or two subjects.

2. In school, is failing several subjects; is one year retarded; doesn't seem to "catch on" to instruction in school; doesn't turn in assignments.

3. Is two or more grades retarded in school; reads more than two grades below grade placement; doesn't get assignments or do any studying on his own.

4. Can't learn well enough to go to regular public or private school.

5. Other (specify) _____

7.   1. In school, has specific complaint about one subject or class, but does attend school almost all the time; feels well when once at school or on job though sometimes objects to going; not upset on return home; occasionally cuts classes or misses work.

2. Often reluctant to go to school or to work; uses any excuse to stay home; claims illness or tends to stay sick longer to remain at home; plays hookey now and then.

3. If forced to go to school or work becomes anxious; has stomach pain; pallor, or trembling; is out of school or work for several weeks at a time with little reason.

4. Absolutely refuses to go to school or work.

5. Other (specify) _____

8. 1. Attention wanders to fantasy when task is especially difficult or tiring; likes to go to room to read; or listens to music; "isolates" self from parents and brothers and sisters when they are near.

2. Prefers to be alone much of the time; has imaginary companions; often lost in thought so that he must be spoken to several times; actively avoids group participation.

3. Has "no friends"; sits and stares for long periods of time; has almost no interests or activities even by self.

4. Lives in world of fantasy; usually confuses fantasy with reality.

5. Other (specify) _____

9. 1. When alone, fears things that are not actually dangerous; has two or three specific fears but is never overcome by fear; doesn't like to be in dark but will for a few moments; fears strangers.

2. Has several specific fears such as animals, bugs, storms, and so on.; becomes so afraid that he (she) refuses temporarily to go outside alone or to school or job; goes out of way to avoid strangers; won't go alone to basement or dark room.

3. Becomes panicked when alone; won't sleep alone in room; panics at sight of strangers, specific objects or animals.

4. Is so fearful that he (she) is too afraid to go to school or job or out of immediate neighborhood.

5. Other (specify) _____

10. 1. Has occasional periods of being afraid or anxious for no apparent reason but he (she) quickly responds to reassurance.

2. Has more frequent or intense periods of fearfulness for no apparent reason and he (she) does not respond readily to reassurance.

3. Is afraid most of the time; often doesn't know or can't say what he fears; is panic-stricken in situations (like storms) far out of proportion to the situation; has sense of impending doom; may express fear of general destruction frequently, or end of world, collapse of home; does not respond to reassurance.

4. Immobilized to point of not being able to leave family because of being afraid; for example, he (she) has feelings of impending doom or destruction or loss of parents or other persons.

5. Other (specify) _____

11.   1. Is slightly fidgety, taps with hands or feet, bites nails, is restless, blushes, perspires; has temporary stage fright when expected to recite for class.

2. Usually fidgety, taps with hands and feet most of time; picks at nose or self; perspires a great deal; bites nails a great deal; gets pale; has difficulty speaking or acting when nervous.

3. Is so nervous that he (she) can't sit still for even a few minutes; can't take examinations or get up to speak in class; is so nervous it is impossible for him (her) to attend school or work.

4. Other (specify) _____

12.   1. Becomes sad if left alone for any length of time; bored easily; once in a while gets moody or mopes around.

2. Complains of unhappiness; often discontented; has the "blues"; complains of being lonely; leaves group to sit on side alone; is not interested in usual entertainment; identifies with lonely animals or persons; cries more than the average person.

3. Does not think much of self; feels he is no good; doesn't want to live; blue or unhappy most of time; so unhappy avoids being with others; threatens suicide; has frequent "accidents."

4. Attempts suicide; so depressed or unhappy that he (she) can't talk or go to school; refuses to get out of bed or leaves his (her) room.

5. Other (specify) _____

13.   1. Suspicious of new foods or places; mild distrust of strangers.

2. Is uncertain about promises being kept; feels people try to fool or trick him; doubts that he (she) is treated fairly; expects to be disappointed; feels that he (she) is being stared at or seriously disapproved of; afraid to trust belongings to care of others.

3. Has fears which result in refusal to go near strange people or away from home; breaks off friendships because of developing suspicions; fears people are out to get or hurt him (her); is certain that he (she) will be disappointed; always expects the worst; thinks there is a "catch" to everything; feels people stare or spy on him (her).

4. Is so distrustful he (she) is unable to have friends; is so distrustful can't carry out everyday activities; suspects other people of actively planning to harm or destroy him (her); becomes panic-striken with distrust; may become violent because of his (her) fear of attack; becomes immobilized because of his suspiciousness.

5. Other (specify) _____

14. 1. Is temporarily disturbed by changes in family routine; does poorly after a change in job, school, or teachers; clings to a few friends and finds it difficult to accept new friends; develops limited play with a few friends.

2. Is openly upset by change in family routine; dreads new situations like new job, teachers, strange places, or meeting new people.

3. Cries or becomes very upset by changes in family routine; seems never to adjust to new schools, new neighborhood, new teacher, or new job.

4. Can't go to new school or take new job; becomes ill about change in routine; won't leave home in new environment or situation.

5. Other (specify)_____

15. 1. Likes to have things prepared in certain ways for sleep or eating; above average in cleanliness and carefulness about dress and self; very polite; desires exact and detailed directions; rarely uses imagination; is only comfortable when the above is done, but can function without.

2. Insists on the set routines above and becomes noticeably upset when these routines fail; becomes irritable when things are not just right, in order, or do not go according to plan; in addition, may have some unusual or unnecessary routine of his own such as putting objects in exact spot, counting them, etc.

3. Has complicated and unnecessary routines which he frequently repeats; if these routines are interfered with, reacts with anger or temper; worries excessively or may become ill; if routines are interfered with some functions such as achievement on job, in school, visiting, or being in groups are interfered with.

4. Needs for his routines are so strong that his basic habits such as eating, sleeping, and so on, cannot be carried on without them, medical care may be required.

5. Other (specify)_____

16. 1. Associates with younger people mainly; avoids leadership even when capable; is slow to assert his (her) rights or opinions; tends to underrate self and abilities.

2. Avoids asserting rights and opinions in situations where it would be to his (her) advantage to do so; dreads taking tests or doesn't do as well on them as he (she) could do; will not compete; feels physically unattractive or unpopular.

3. Goes to extreme (e.g., walks many blocks to avoid threat of fight or stays home); failing at school in spite of adequate intelligence; won't hand in assignments because of fear of failure; convinced he (she) is not good enough; feels unloved.

4. Overwhelmed by feeling inferior to the extent that he (she) avoids all social situations, will not leave home alone, will not go to school.

5. Other (specify) _____

17. 1. Sometimes acts before he thinks but only in situations in which results are not serious; is careless; acts hastily with siblings or close friends but can withhold his actions if necessary.

2. Has difficulty controlling feelings; gets angry easily; gives possessions away or takes things away without thinking; often acts before he (she) thinks; reacts with excitement to minor events.

3. Loses control of impulses; can't tell from one moment to another what he (she) is going to do; can't be trusted to act without supervision; sets fires; hits others without provocation; often endangers self or others, for example, drives a car recklessly; satisfies own needs immediately and without thought.

4. Difficulty in controlling behavior is so extreme that he (she) must be restrained for own and other's safety and/or protection of property.

5. Other (specify) _____

18. 1. Becomes irritable when provoked; complains and whines; "sasses back" when corrected or ordered to do something.

2. Gets very angry; kicks and hits at others; frequently screams when can't have his (her) own way; has angry outbursts against others; throws articles in anger.

3. Gets so angry that he (she) becomes unconscious for a moment; holds breath in anger; violent attacks on others; hurts self; becomes so angry that he (she) destroys important property.

4. Temper displays are so serious that he must be confined or restrained, for safety of self and others; goes out of his (her) head.

5. Other (specify) _____

19. 1. Pouts; minor resistance to rules and regulations; sulking; slow to get work done; puts off tasks.

2. Frequently resists any rules and regulations; sullen and unresponsive to the point of avoiding requirements; prolonged dawdling in all daily activities on job, at school, and at home; uses conversation to avoid tasks; fails to follow rules and does something else without openly refusing.

3. Sullenly refuses to do what is required; openly does the opposite of what is required.

4. Refuses to respond to requests; won't talk, eat, urinate, or have bowel movements, and so forth.

5. Other (specify) _____

20. 1. Tells a fib or exaggerates now and then; tells a small lie to escape punishment or to inflate his (her) own accomplishments.

2. Frequently tells a lie when confronted with misbehavior and/or to build self up; often deceives parents or spouse as to where he (she) has been; says he (she) hasn't homework when he (she) has, and so on.

3. Lies most of the time; apparently would rather tell a lie than the truth.

4. Lies so frequently and seriously that he (she) has no friends; is totally untrustworthy.

5. Other (specify) _____

21. 1. Takes a few cents once in a while; if temptation is especially strong will take something of small value; occasionally picks up something in a store.

2. Takes money which is seen as a substantial amount; takes objects once in a while and does not tend to return them; will keep change unless parents specifically ask for it.

3. Steals frequently valuable property such as automobile accessories, automobiles, expensive jewelry; may use threats or force in stealing; enters homes or business establishments to steal.

4. Steals so frequently and such valuable property that must be constantly watched, e.g., can't work where stealing is possible. Court action may or may not be involved.

5. Other (specify) _____

22. 1. Masturbates and/or touches sex organs but infrequently and when there is nothing else to do; wants to examine other peoples' bodies; dresses or behaves in a "sexy" way; wants to date early.

2. Frequently masturbates at home or occasionally at school; sex curiosity about others makes others keep away from him (her); likes

to take enemas; very interested in sex organs of persons or animals; early petting or necking; excessive interest in sexually stimulating movies or literature; is easily aroused sexually.

3. Openly masturbates in public; attempts to look at others' sex organs; has sexual relations with others of same sex or with animals; has frequent sexual activity with person of opposite sex; is constantly attending sexually stimulating movies and reading sexually stimulating literature.

4. Is completely rejected because of sex behavior; can't attend school because of sex behavior; sex misbehavior is so extreme that confinement is a present or constant threat.

5. Other (specify) _____

23. 1. Overly familiar with any and all strangers; has strange likes and dislikes such as food fads and clothing fads; strange behavior such as rubbing surfaces, unusual interest in smelling objects; excessive interest in insects, animals, space, or other peculiar intellectual interests.

2. Has continuous interest and occupation with unusual things and subjects; often does not hear; seems lost in thought when spoken to; talks to self even when others are near; scratches self or picks at self; wanders away alone and at odd hours.

3. Displays feelings that seem to have no cause and/or would seem wrong for the situation, such as uncontrollable giggling, crying; speaks without making sense; makes strange noises; becomes completely involved with peculiar things such as specks of dust, distant sounds; hurts self on purpose or tries to destroy self; frequently insists on extremely unusual dress habits; has very odd habits such as tapping self for long periods of time; has hallucinations (sees or hears things that are not there), delusions (has beliefs that are entirely at odds with reality and cannot be convinced they are wrong).

4. Can't attend school or work because of strange and unacceptable behavior; needs institutionalization or constant supervision because of this behavior.

5. Other (specify) _____

24. 1. Fails to do school work as an expression of resistance to authority; sometimes lies to parents to cover up; has few or no friends because of his treating them badly, argues occasionally with adults; can easily excuse himself or avoid tasks with "fast talking"; resists the responsibility of going to school but does it; stays out late at night without planned activity.

2. Sometimes skips school or work to do other things; frequently lies but obeys if forced to do so; defies authority; joins gangs for the purpose of rebellion against authorities; steals, destroys property; is cruel to animals; does "bad" adult things such as early smoking, spending much time hanging around places of commercial recreation meant only for adults (e.g., pool halls, burlesque shows, taverns); runs away from home for hours at a time; on a few occasions has had sexual relations.

3. Frequently skips school or work; lies a great deal; actively participates in such gang activities as cruelty, attacks on people, robbery and so on; stays out all night or nearly all night without permission; frequently has sex relations outside marriage.

4. Expelled from school or in danger of being expelled because of behavior; in prison or reform school because of delinquent (antisocial) behavior.

5. Other (specify) _____

25. 1. Asks for slightly more help than usual for his age; likes to go with mother around house; asks teacher or boss several times about instructions.

2. Asks frequently to be helped at home and at school or on job; tries to push brothers and sisters aside to get mother's or father's attention; spends most of recreation time with parents; won't let parents talk to company without butting in; usually won't start activities on his own.

3. Needs constant urging and reassurance; never lets mother out of sight when at home; is constantly center of attention, otherwise unhappy; constantly accuses parents of favoring brothers and sisters; extremely dependent upon parents for help in carrying out basic daily functions and school work.

4. Cannot function without adult's help; so dependent that cannot marry, get job, attend school or make any of own decisions.

5. Other (specify) _____

26. 1. Has few friends; difficulty in adjusting to the group's activities; doesn't stick up for self enough; sometimes lets others take unfair advantage of him to moderate degree; is shy around opposite sex.

2. Associates only with younger people; is a bully or often complains of being bullied; avoids or becomes very anxious around the opposite sex.

3. No friends through all life except casual acquaintances; always feels unwanted; actively avoids being with others (e.g., school groups); actively rejected by both sexes.

4. Must stay at home or has no social life because of being overly aggressive or having fear of failure.

5. Other (specify) _____

27. 1. Has trouble with parents at home; seems fearful and shy around adults; sometimes willful and disobedient to parents; ignores parents on occasion; tends to get along better with one sex of adult; interferes with parents' social life; whines, can't care for self according to age.

2. Has trouble with adults at home and at school; seems excessively rude to adults; often unmanageable; parents and teacher often "can't get through" to him; much prefers one sex of adult; demands constant attention and supervision.

3. Trouble extreme with adults outside home; looks down on parents as inferiors; flatly refuses to obey; has almost no reasonable relationship with adults; takes over one parent's role; for example, mother-son-relationship, rejecting father; extremely close; demands time, feeding, love, direction, and constant supervision.

4. Is so difficult to manage that parents seriously consider having him institutionalized; can't attend school or get job because of fear of teachers or because is so disobedient, unruly, irresponsible, rebellious, and so on.

5. Other (specify) _____

28. 1. Slow in activities that call for coordination (motor skills); clumsiness.

2. Poorly coordinated; can't catch ball; very poor in sports; can't ride a bicycle; has many falls; mild tremors or spasticity; gets very tense or shakes when he (she) tries to do tasks calling for coordination.

3. Cerebral palsy, spastic; serious defects in coordination and motor functions (e.g., walking, balance); falls very often; can't write because of poor motor coordination; severe tremors.

4. Can't move without help because of nerve and/or muscular disability.

5. Other (specify) _____

29. 1. Mildly restless; moves around on chairs; doesn't like activities that require sitting still.

2. Restless, won't stay put; constantly fidgets; swings legs or moves arms; sleeps "all over the bed."

3. Is unable to remain in school or on job full day because of restlessness; paces floor; talks excessively; so restless can sleep only a few hours at night.

    4. So active is harmful to self or others; must be restrained; can't attend school or work because of it.

    5. Other (specify) _____

30. 1. Occasionally because of poor planning gets into dangerous situations of a mild nature (e.g., bumping head, tripping, minor cuts); has more accidents than the usual person.

    2. Does not take ordinary precautions where danger is seen; in spite of caution, manages to have accidents of moderate degree (e.g., breaking bones, bicycles); can't use ordinary tools (e.g., scissors to cut with, hammer) because of danger of hurting self; eats and drinks harmful substances.

    3. Persistently runs or rushes headlong into very dangerous situations (e.g., busy streets, very high places, path of fast moving vehicles); eats or drinks things in container clearly marked as dangerous.

    4. Because of the above behavior, has crippled or seriously injured self; requires constant supervision, can't be alone in yard or go to school alone; has frequently been to the hospital because of injuries.

    5. Other (specify) _____

31. 1. Occasionally complains of stomachaches when tense or upset.

    2. Frequently complains of stomach pains; has nausea or vomits; has trouble swallowing; has diarrhea; has important food "allergies"; is underdeveloped or slightly overweight.

    3. Has frequent pain in stomach; serious weight loss; serious diarrhea or ulcerative colitis; internal bleeding; gastric ulcer; very thin or markedly obese.

    4. Because of the above characteristics, is now or should be hospitalized.

    5. Other (specify) _____

32. 1. Has complaints of joint pains or muscle weakness or headaches as a common response to illness or tension.

    2. Frequently has complaints of symptoms such as joint pains, weakness, fainting or dizziness, numbness or paralysis, frequent headaches.

    3. Has serious complaints such as arthritis, wasting disease of the nervous system; recurring epilepsy; has persistent long-lasting paralysis.

    4. Is now or should be hospitalized for the above symptoms.

    5. Other (specify) _____

33. 1. Complains of slight trouble in seeing, hearing, or peculiar sensations but only when due to illness or extreme nervousness.

2. Frequently has complaints of poor, double, or peculiar vision; ringing in ears or poor hearing.

3. Is partially or totally blind or deaf or has a serious defect in any other sense.

4. Blindness, deafness, and so on, prevents working or attendance at any school or creates conditions of total dependency on others.

5. Other (specify) _____

34. 1. Stutters slightly (about 2% of words); omits, substitutes, or distorts sounds but speech is understandable; voice is different from those his (her) own age—nasal, too loud, too soft; sometimes has difficulty understanding what is said to him and in expressing ideas even though hearing is normal.

2. Stutters noticeably (about 5 to 8% of words); stuttering accompanied by distracting sounds and facial movements; omits, substitutes, or distorts sounds to such a degree that speech is distorted; voice varies in such a way, being too loud, soft, nasal, high-pitched, that it calls attention to itself; often has difficulty understanding what is said to him (her) and in expressing ideas even though hearing is normal.

3. Stutters a great deal (about 12 to 25% of words); stuttering accompanied by distracting facial gestures, movements of the body, arms or legs, and distracting sounds; omits, substitutes, or distorts sounds to such a degree that speech is not understandable; voice varies so much from what one would expect that speech is often not understandable; comprehends little of what is said to him (her) and does not use speech as a main means of communication even though hearing is normal.

4. Speech disorder is so severe that speech is not understandable and therefore cannot be used as the means of communication.

5. Other (specify) _____

35. 1. Has complaints of trouble urinating or frequently has pain when urinating at times of illness or other nervousness.

2. Frequently has complaints of symptoms such as pain or trouble urinating, genitals did not develop properly.

3. Has serious complaints or symptoms such as repeated urinary infections, kidney disease, genitals obviously defective, bladder defective, has had surgical treatment.

4. Because of the above difficulties, has had prolonged hospitalization.

5. Other (specify) _____

36. 1. Has complaints of trouble breathing or coughing or hiccoughs in response to illness or extreme nervousness; has frequent colds.

2. Has frequent coughing, wheezing, or asthma or shortness of breath on exertion; often has sinus trouble, flu, bronchitis, tonsilitis; has had pneumonia.

3. Has persistent asthma or pneumonia or bronchitis, tuberculosis, or other serious respiratory disease.

4. Because of the above disorders, has had prolonged hospitalization or confinement in bed at home.

5. Other (specify) _____

37. 1. Complains of chest pain, pounding heart, or coldness of hands and feet, or gets very pale when ill or extremely nervous.

2. Complains frequently of chest pain, pounding heart, persistent coldness of hands or feet, mild heart murmurs, mild shortness of breath while playing or active in sports.

3. Has heart defect or disease; persistent shortness of breath even when physical activity is limited or when the least bit upset.

4. No physical exercise, work, or school attendance allowed by physician because of heart defect; has required hospitalization because of the above characteristics.

5. Other (specify) _____

38. 1. Is a little behind others his age in understanding what is said to him, following directions, remembering things, concentrating on or solving a problem.

2. Is a year or so behind other children in understanding what is said to him, following directions, or remembering things, concentrating on or solving a problem.

3. Must be constantly watched so that he (she) does not endanger self or others.

4. Is unable to do any of above things; is bedridden and needs custodial care.

5. Other (specify) _____

DIAGNOSTIC GUIDELINES

Clinical Diagnosis of Child

These are not exhaustive descriptions of each diagnostic category. They are highlights and are meant as reminders.

1. Normal

In spite of current manifest behavior disturbances the personality growth is essentially healthy and falls within the wide range of "variations of normality."

2. Transient or Developmental Problems

In this classification reactions are more or less transient in character and appear to be an acute symptom response to a situation without apparent underlying personality disturbance. There is no previous history that would indicate more extreme psychopathology is involved. It includes age appropriate developmental strains (e.g., negativism at 2 years of age, expression of sexual feelings at 5 years, emancipation from parents as a teenager). It also takes in transient reactions to physical handicaps, ill health, moving, hospitalization, and so forth. In the presence of good adaptive capacity, recession of symptoms generally occurs when the situational stress diminishes.

3. Neurotic Reaction

In these reactions internalized conflicts and anxiety dominate the clinical picture. Anxiety may be directly felt or expressed or be unconsciously and automatically controlled by the utilization of various defense mechanisms. There is no evidence of gross disorganization of the personality.

4. Neurotic Behavior Disorder

In this reaction there is a significant admixture of external and internalized conflict with some indication that guilt and/or anxiety is present through superego manifestation. There appears to be potential for reversing the regression that has taken place.

5. Character Disorder

In this reaction anxiety is minimized or absent or anxiety occurs only in the face of punishment. It is a heterogeneous category of developmental defects with pathological trends in the personality structure. It very often reflects life-long interpersonal conflict manifested as habitual, standardized and inflexible modes of response. Character disturbances are limitations or pathological forms of treating the external world, internal drives, and demands of the superego. The disturbance is lifelong and ego syntonic. The primary characteristics of this reaction are 1) habitual and inflexible modes of behavior, 2) lack of anxiety or psychological discomfort, 3) behavior often provoking dislike and concern in others, 4) ego syntonic, lifelong disturbance pattern, 5) failure to learn from experience.

6. Borderline Psychosis

In this classification there is an intermittent loss of contact with reality but with recoverability. There is a tenuous hold on or contact with reality. It is also characterized by such behavior as fixed obsessions, bizarre fantasies, peculiar, unusual behavior, low frustration tolerance, emotional immaturity, unevenness of development, periodic impulse breakthrough, poor judgment, and/or neurotic and somatic traits. Other features of this reaction are deficiencies of object relations, inability to tolerate heightened stimulation, and withdrawal from reality at the slightest provocation.

7. Psychotic Reaction

There is a loss of contact with and withdrawal from reality and bizarre, peculiar fantasies and behavior. A multiplicity of signs may be present such as: lack of spontaneity, bizarre motor hyperactivity, dissociated movements, disturbances of motor coordination, poor control, overwhelming anxiety about body image, disorientation in time and space, unusual sensitivity to sensory stimulation, excessive vulnerability to emotional hurt, violent expressions of emotion. In addition, there is typically an unevenness in intellectual development and function, failure to differentiate between animate and inanimate objects, extreme dependency on one adult, much greater attachment to toys or pet animals than to human associates, and extreme withdrawal and autism. In this reaction there are marked arrests, unevenness and regressions of ego and superego development with crippling effects on personality growth and symptom formation.

8. Mental Deficiency

This reaction includes deficiencies of an organic and/or functional nature as a result of a multiplicity of causes, i.e., heredity, metabolic disorder, organic damage, or environmental distortions which retard intellectual and cognitive development with resultant and concomitant personality limitations and distortions.

9. Brain Syndrome

This syndrome has the following typical signs: hyperactivity, distractibility, poor attention span, low frustration tolerance with exaggerated reaction, visual-motor deficits, language and communication impairment leading to poorly integrated and unpredictable behavior. There may be a concomitant personality distortion, particularly awareness or a concern regarding a perceived difference from normal and etiology may be congenital, hereditary, infectious, traumatic, and so forth.

10. Psychophysiological Disorder

Syndrome by present theory associated with personality or emotional disorders or symptoms which are due to a chronic and exaggerated state of the normal physiological expression of emotion with the feeling being repressed (e.g., ulcerative colitis, asthma, anorexia nervosa, ulcers, hypertension).

APPENDIX B

Forms for Rating Childhood Data

The same Social Adjustment Rating form was used to rate both childhood data and adult social adjustment at follow-up. For brevity, the Parental Adjustment Rating Form is presented with items covered, but not the pre-coded categories. Psychiatric and psychological data were rated at follow-up, but were based on clinic data obtained in childhood. The same items were rated by both psychiatrists and psychologists. Only excerpts from the Manual for Psychological Ratings are included here for illustrative purposes.

SOCIAL ADJUSTMENT RATINGS

Underline phrase that applies; write in additional ones. Circle rating. 1=good; 2=mild maladjustment; 3=moderate maladjustment; 4=serious maladjustment; 5=incapacitating. For each rating, circle (one) degree of certainty: +=you are very sure of your rating; 0=you are not very sure or have sparse data; −=you are not at all sure or have insufficient data.

A. Within Family (+, 0, −)

1. Gets along well with other family members; is well liked by them and likes them; identifies with parent of same sex without being too close or conforming; can talk to parents and work out disagreements; no problems.

2. Somewhat unhappy; not as well-liked as other members of the family; feels he is picked on; argues with siblings or parents; sometimes starts fights; sometimes resists discipline; moody now and then; dawdles or resists family plans; doesn't stand up for self; a little too eager to please, conform.

3. Often keeps to self; stays in room quite a bit or watches TV for hours as a way of excluding others; accuses others in family of not trusting him; once in a while takes something that doesn't belong to him; lies to get out of trouble; fights quite a bit with siblings; sasses parents; cries when disciplined or frustrated; stays away from home hours at a

233

time; wants more than his share of goods or privileges; stubborn; jealous of siblings; too dependent on parents; refuses to share. For adults: has experimented with marijuana or liquor; feels he is restricted.

4. Very isolated, rarely communicates with others in family; constantly disagrees with them and almost always resists family plans or breaks family rules; cruel; physically attacks others even when unprovoked; yells and swears at parents; often disregards personal rights or property of others; cries frequently, often without apparent reason; talks about suicide; starts small fires but none serious to safety of family; runs away from home overnight or for weekend but comes back on own. For adults: drinks frequently; frequently uses marijuana, has experimented with "hard" drugs; still living at home past 22; still has only his family for companionship; extremely stubborn; very dependent on parents or siblings, hates for them to be gone, wants to "tag along." For child: has experimented with marijuana or alcohol; extremely stubborn.

5. So withdrawn he can't be reached; so negativistic he is no longer a part of the family planning; does serious bodily harm to others in the family so that he has to be watched and restrained; has no sense of others' rights or property; has made serious suicide attempts; is a drug addict; is an alcoholic; adjustment within family so poor that he had to be removed from family; can't be away from parents for more than a few hours.

B. School and/or Job Performance (+, 0, −)

1. Working at expected or advanced grade level; good study habits; does work efficiently and promptly; is creative and imaginative in his work; gets regular promotions; finished high school and is in, or is fairly sure to go to, college; for adults: has steady job and is doing well in it.

2. Is at grade level but achieving below grade level in one or two subjects (not failing any); occasionally doesn't do homework; difficulty in concentrating but gets work done. Gets job done but not as well as other workers; has had only a few (1 to 3) failing grades in all of school history, does very well in subjects he likes, less well in others.

3. May be one grade behind; failing one or two subjects; all-around achievement not up to capacity; rarely studies, neglects homework; difficulty in concentration affects grades; has had numerous failing grades in school history; is criticized on job for not doing work properly but is able to keep job; feels inadequate at times on job; is late

to work occasionally; has had to go to summer school at least once to keep up; is in college but unable to carry a full load because of grades; went to special school; in danger of dropping out of school or having to transfer because of failure.

4. More than one grade behind; having to transfer because of failure to measure up; can't get into college because of poor grades although he has the ability; has dropped out of school for a year or more; changes jobs or gets fired frequently for poor performance; often out of work; can't get the job he wants; hates his work but has to keep it because of money; is often absent from work.

5. Has dropped out of school; dismissed because of failure to achieve or inability to concentrate. Can't hold a job at all.

C. Relationship to Teachers or Boss (+, 0, −)

1. Gets along well with teacher or boss; enjoys participating in classwork and activities; offers to help others.

2. Dawdles in doing work; inattentive at times; mildly disobedient or resistive to rules; compliant but doesn't relate in positive way; ingratiates self to gain favor.

3. Occasionally sullen and negativistic; talks back to teacher or boss; tends to reject teacher's or boss's offer of help; needs much instruction or help in order to function; "polishes the apple;" once in a while is "called on the carpet" at work or sent to principal's office; doesn't relate to teachers or boss except when absolutely necessary.

4. So sullen or negativistic that teacher or boss actively dislikes him and is considering his transfer or dismissal; does so little that he can't be promoted; is often sent to principal's office or to higher authority; strikes out physically at those in authority; so withdrawn or isolated he may not be able to continue; has been temporarily suspended from school or job; feels boss or teachers "pick" on him, treat others better than him; refuses to discuss problems about school or boss.

5. Has been expelled or permanently dismissed; quit job because he couldn't take orders or get along with others.

D. Relationship to Peers (+, 0, −)

1. Well-liked and participates in many peer activities; can seek out others and others seek him out for companionship or for help; has friends of both sexes; late adolescence: has one *best* friend of opposite sex and at least one of same sex.

2. Has a little difficulty initiating friendships but can respond to others; a little domineering or selfish but most of the time gets along well; has a few close friends but not a wide circle of friends; tends to avoid organized activities; more comfortable with younger or less adequate individuals; dislikes other young people who are different from himself.

3. Has trouble in making or accepting friendships; is shy; withdraws if criticized; sometimes drives friends temporarily away by being selfish or bossy; lets others take advantage of him; prefers younger or less adequate friends; lets others make decisions for him; yells at peers; frequently picks fights. For young child: prefers only children of opposite sex; frequently changes friends.

4. Is a loner; so withdrawn or so domineering that he has only one friend or no friend; rarely takes part in social activities; interacts minimally or excludes interaction with one of the sexes altogether; interacts exclusively with younger or less adequate people; attacks verbally and/or physically in serious ways; relates to only one sex as friend; has no interest in marrying; wants to join armed services to escape present acquaintances.

5. No contact with peers at all except in hospital or other institution; may be completely isolated at home.

E. Relationships in Larger Society (+, 0, —)

1. For child: takes part in neighborhood activities, scouts, clubs, church. For adult: takes part in community activities such as church, social organizations, political activities; votes if old enough to do so, etc.; volunteers services to needy.

2. Gets along fairly well in community but is not an active participant in groups or organizations of constructive or recreational nature; goes "along with rules" and regulations passively.

3. For adults: has been stopped "on suspicion" at least once by police; has been arrested for minor law violations (truancy, vagrancy, etc.) or once for major violation (theft, attack, drug abuse, etc.). Takes no interest in community activities of constructive nature; has been intoxicated in public and had to be brought home. For child: is a loner; seeks isolated interests; is somewhat secretive; trouble maker in the neighborhood or other group; belongs to a destructive gang; occasional truancy.

4. For child: has been in trouble with police (e.g., has been stopped on suspicion, brought home by police); was suspended from school for several days to one week; experimented with drugs and/or alcohol; prolonged truancy (over 1 week or frequently); occasional running away from home. For adults: has been in trouble with the law more than once; was hospitalized or in treatment center for six months or

less; was in jail or reformatory for overnight or longer; belongs to a rebel organization; takes part in riots or gang fights; has been hospitalized overnight or longer for drugs.

5. For child: can't stay in own home; should be placed in correctional institution or inpatient treatment center. For adult: is in prison or reformatory; hospitalized now or spent more than six months in hospital or other closed institution; has "dropped out" and no longer relates to family or friends.

F. Overall Rating of Life Adjustment (Functioning) (+, 0, −)

1. Has functioned well at home, in school, on job (according to his ability). At home: gets along as well as most children do; no serious authority or discipline problems; gets along with peers; has friends appropriate to age level. Life shows purpose. Is reasonably happy, content. No psychiatric or other referral since he was here.

2. Somewhat unhappy; mild problems either in nervousness, bothersome habits, minor acting out but attends school regularly; keeps a job; no brush with law; may have had a recommendation for psychiatric treatment or one contact with law agency. (Mild neurotic, mild character problem, habit disturbance.)

3. Is singled out in school as a poor student, or socially inept, or both, but is able to stay in school, or hold a job. May have had short-term outpatient psychiatric or other treatment or one contact with law agency. Isn't happy; not achieving up to capacity; only a few friends. (Neurotic or moderate character disorders; not psychotic or psychopathic.)

4. Was hospitalized for six months or less and/or was under intensive psychiatric or other psychological treatment or should be (it was recommended several times); recurrent contact with the law; school attendance very poor; two or more grades behind in school; can't get along with peers; can't keep friends. (Seriously neurotic, sociopathic, borderline psychosis.)

5. Hospitalized or in prison now. Can't function as independent adult; needs supervision. Incapacitated as far as steady work or school; may be at home now but not functioning independently. (Severe borderline psychosis, psychosis, psychopath.)

PARENTAL ADJUSTMENT RATINGS

(To be coded from childhood social history and intake)

1. *Parents' Reaction to Child*
   (*present* parents in household unless otherwise stated).

A. Was child wanted by mother (natural mother)?

B. Was child wanted by father (natural father)?

C. Mother's feeling about child (at time of clinic service).

D. Father's feeling about child (at time of clinic service).

E. Does either (or both) parent(s) see in this child someone else, for example, his/her sister, brother, aunt, uncle, mgm, mgf, pgm, pgf, other (mother, father, both)?

F. Mother disciplines child reasonably or inconsistently.

G. Father disciplines child reasonably or inconsistently.

H. Discipline is consistent between parents.

 I. Parents' reaction to child's problem.

J. Parents' relationship to each other.

K. Mother's emotional stability.

L. Father's emotional stability.

M. Mother's capacity to cope under stress.

N. Father's capacity to cope under stress.

O. Early trauma (in first 5 years), especially separation, loss, hospitalization.

P. Evidence for possible organic damage (prenatal, perinatal, postnatal, infant, and child).

MANUAL FOR RATINGS FROM PSYCHOLOGICAL EVALUATION

Specific Indices of Disturbance

Adequacy of Thought Processes and Disturbance (rate 1 to 5 on each).

1. Thinking (logicality)

1 = logical cause and effect relationships in TAT stories, Comprehension subtest, Rorschach: lack of confabulation, contamination, fabulized combination, etc.

2 = one instance, only, of outright loose thinking in whole test battery or a few *tendencies* toward illogical or alogical thinking but only on Rorschach.

3 = a few (2 or 3) instances of loose thinking on Rorschach with some difficulty in recovery; WISC and TAT quite logical.

4 = several (4 or over) instances of primary process thinking including some bizarreness, confabulation, contamination, including some loss of logic and/or fluidity in TAT and/or WISC.

[a]Scale points avilable but not included here.

5 = *All* tests characterized by fluidity, bizarreness, illogicality, primary process, etc.

2. *Reality Testing*[a]

3. *Concreteness*[a]

4. *Degree of Anxiety* (Anxiety as shown by constriction, segmentation, etc., should also be rated)

1 = optimal anxiety; mild but appropriate anxiety where stimulus definitely calls for it.

2 = mild anxiety in connection with a central conflict with quick recovery; for example, one or two anxious Rorschach responses; Digit Span and timed tests a little lower than other subtests.

3 = moderate anxiety as shown by a few shading responses, or several percepts of anxious content (clouds, ghosts, anatomy, etc.), color shock and long reaction time to a few cards, slight intratest and intertest variability, *or* anxiety lacking in cards where it would be expected.

4 = severe: rapid breakdown in Rorschach in terms of loss of accuracy in the area of conflict, slow recovery after an anxious percept, much shading, blocking in Rorschach and in TAT, rejection of one or more projective stimuli, great intratest and intertest variability, *or* evidence of anxiety almost absent even where stimulus should evoke it.

5 = incapacitating anxiety so that testing was nearly impossible or had to be terminated before completion; no anxiety whatsoever shown.

5. *Object Relations*[a]

6. *Identity*[a]

7. *Superego*[a]

8. *Emotionality*[a]

9. *Aggressiveness*[a]

10. a) *Major Conflicts*[a]
    b) *Defenses*[a]

11. *Coping*

1 = subject poses problems in TAT that are realistic for his age level and solves them constructively and in socially acceptable ways; reasonable and practical solutions in Comprehension and Picture Arrangement subtests; Rorschach shows integrative level expected of age.

[a]Scale points available but not included here.

2 = one or two destructive, impractical, or improbable solutions in TAT; some "1" answers in Comprehension at age level in subtest.

3 = about one-fourth of TAT stories have destructive, impractical or improbable solutions; moderately poor Comprehension and Picture Arrangement solutions for age level.

4 = half of TAT stories have destructive, impractical or improbable solutions; several instances of Wishful Thinking; Comprehension and/or Picture Arrangement are among lowest of his subtest scores.

5 = TAT stories are almost entirely lacking in practical, socially acceptable solutions; several may have no solutions at all.

12. *Pathology of Content*[a]

[a] Scale points available but not included here.

APPENDIX C

Forms for Follow-Up Data and Reliability

GUIDELINES

Check one: Subject about self: ( ) Mother about subject: ( )

Name: _____

Date: _____

Age: _____

INTERVIEWER: _____

1. Are you married? Yes___ No___

   a. Age when married___

   b. First marriage Yes___ No___: Number___

2. Do you have children?

   a. Yes___ Ages and Sex _____

   b. No___

3. Living with:

   a. Spouse___

   b. Parents___ Siblings age and sex___

   c. Roommate___ Sex___

   d. Alone___

4. (For Mother)

   How many children do you have?_____

   a. Ages and sex _____

   b. Have you had any other children that needed special help? _____

   c. Why? _____

   Special School? _____

   Hospitalized? _____

   When? _____

   How long? _____

    d. Is he (she) living at home now? _____

      If not, where? _____

      For how long? _____

5. Number of changes in residence in past 10 years _____

6. School:

    a. Grade completed ____

    b. Average grades ____ Dropped out? Yes ___ No ___

    c. Major field of interest _____

7. What is your occupation? _____

    a. Part time ____ where _____

    b. Full time ____ where _____

    c. Ever fired from a job? ____

    d. If yes, why? _____

8. Describe physical health:

    a. Robust ____ b. Average ____ c. Poor ____

9. Medication

    a. Yes ___

    b. No ___

    c. If yes, what kind? _____

10. Have you ever been hospitalized overnight?

    a. Yes ____ Why? _____

    b. No ___

    c. Attempted suicide? _____

11. Have you ever been in trouble with the law?

    a. If yes, why? _____

    b. Convicted: Yes ___ No ___

    c. Jailed: Yes ___ No ___ d. If yes, how long? _____

12. Have you ever used drugs?

    a. Yes ___ b. No ___ c. If yes, what kind? _____

    d. How often? *(write in type)*

      Within last 6 mos.   Prior to 6 mos.

13. Do you use liquor?

a. Yes___ b. No___ c. If yes, what kind?_____

d. How often?

14. Have you needed any help such as AA? *(Explain)*

15. Are you in the service now?

    a. Yes___ b. No___ c. Reserves?___

    d. If yes, what branch?

    e. If discharged, Honorable?___

               Dishonorable?___

               Other?___ Why?_____

16. (Subject only)

(For interviewer: record during or *right after* interview)

    a. Seems anxious, nervous, worried? Yes___ No___ *(Describe)*

    b. Seems to present self openly, or seems to present self in "good light"?

    c. Tells about something unhappy or painful, and then denies it later or denies feeling anything about it?
Or sees all of life as (unrealistically) troublefree? *(Describe)*

    d. Tends to blame others for his misfortunes or inadequacies? *(Describe)*

    e. Describes strict adherence to order and extreme carefulness, cleanliness, etc.? *(Describe)*

    f. Talks about very primitive impulses and experiences without any inhibition (e.g., sexual experiences, aggression)? *(Describe)*

    g. What kinds of emotion did the subject display in the interview? *(Describe)*
What kinds did subject tell about in relation to past experiences? *(Describe)*
Do these seem appropriate to the situation? Yes___ No___ Explain.
Was subject able to control this emotion?_____ —End it and go on with other material?_____

    h. Seems to trust interviewer? Yes___ No___
If no, then how intensive is the distrust? *(Describe)*
In describing relationships with others, seemed able to trust, or suspicious, reserved, self-centered, etc. *(Describe)*
Seems to have a sense of right and wrong?
Respects the rights of others even if he didn't like them?
Cares about others? *(Describe)*

Essay Section

17. Tell me about school (work).

    How did you get along with the teachers (boss)?

    What subjects you liked and didn't like.

    What clubs you belonged to.

18. Tell me how you get along with your brothers and sisters.

    Do you share a room?

    Is there one you like (dislike) more than the others?   Why?

    What do you do with your brothers and sisters?

19. Tell me how you get along with your parents.

    Are you closer to one than the other?

    Are they fair in their treatment of you?

    Do they discipline you? If so, how?

    What kinds of things do you do with them?

    Can you talk things over with mother? With father?

20. Tell me how you get along with your spouse.

    What do you do together?

    Do you have secrets from each other?

    If children—what do you do with them? To take care of them?

    Do you have disagreements?

21. Tell me about your friends.

    Do you date? How often?

    What do you like about dating?

    How many friends do you have?

    How often do you see your friends?

    How long have you known your best friends?

    What sex is your best friend?

22. Have you seen any mental health worker since the clinic?

    Tell me about it.

23. Do you remember coming to the clinic?

    Why did you come?

    Whom did you see?

    Did it help you? Explain.

24. How do you feel about yourself?

    Are you happy?

    Adjusting to life?

25. Have there been any crises in your life since the clinic?

    Tell me about them.

26. What would you change about your life?

    Do you think you'll marry someday? Why?

    Is there anything you would like to tell me?

RELIABILITY OF THE RATINGS

Reliability of judgmental ratings was assessed 1) through having two professionals each make independent ratings from recorded materials, that is, psychological test protocols, psychiatric interview process typescripts, intake and social history recordings, and interview forms and typescripts from follow-up contacts and 2) through having two professionals interview a follow-up subject together and make their ratings independently. In the first procedure, two social workers made Social Adjustment, Personal Adjustment, and Parental Ratings from the intake and social history information put into the chart at the time of the clinic diagnostic; two psychologists, using childhood test protocols, made ratings on 12 personality variables and a global rating of severity of disturbance and two psychiatrists, using psychiatric interview typescripts, rated the same variables. In the second procedure, the two interviewers independently rated Social Adjustment and Personal Adjustment after their joint follow-up interview of the subject and, separately, of his mother.

Ratings of Childhood Data

1. Social Adjustment, Personal Adjustment, and Parental Ratings.

Two social workers rated 15 cases on these forms, using the 5-point scale defined for each item. On the first five items of the Social Adjustment form (adjustment in family, in school or job, to teachers or boss, to peers and in larger society), out of the total 73 judgments made, the two social workers made exactly the same rating in 54 (74%), were one step apart in 17 ratings (23%), and 2 steps apart in only 2 (3%) of the judgments. (Two of the total 75 items could not be rated because one child was not in school.)

In rating of overall social adjustment (Item F), the two social workers agreed on 13 of the 15 children and were one step apart on the other two.

The same 15 cases and the same two social workers were used to assess interrater agreement on Personal Adjustment. Of 88 judgments made, the two raters agreed on 67, or 76%, were one step apart on the 5-step scale on 20, or 23%, and two steps apart on one judgment (1%).

Agreement on 16 variables having to do with parents' relationship, stability, and so forth, and their feelings toward this child for the 15 cases was also computed. Ratings could be made on 217 of a possible 240 items. The two social workers agreed on 160, or 74%, of these 217 ratings, were one step apart on 45, or 21%, and two steps apart on 12, or 5%, of the total.

2. Psychological ratings from childhood test data.

A pair of psychologists, using intelligence and projective personality test protocols from the subjects' childhood, independently assessed 6 children on 12 personality variables and rated them as to overall severity of disturbance. On 72 ratings of personality, there was exact agreement on 51, or 71%, a one-step difference on 20, or 28%, and a two-step difference on the one remaining rating. Exact agreement on the overall severity of disturbance was shown in 5 of the 6 cases and the ratings of severity on the sixth child were one step apart.

Ratings at follow-up

1. Social Adjustment ratings.

Two interviewers, working together, saw 11 subjects and their mothers. Percent of agreement was calculated between pairs of interviewers on these cases with one interviewer taking part in all 11 cases and paired with 6 other interviewers. Percent of agreement on the 55 items representing 5 areas of adjustment on the 11 young adults was as follows: 31, or 56%, of the ratings were identical; 21, or 38%, were one step apart; and 3, or 5%, were 2 steps apart. Interrater reliability was also computed for the sum of these five items (ASSA); $r = .78$.

The paired ratings of overall adjustment (ALAR) for these 11 subjects agreed exactly in 7 cases (64%) and were one step apart in the other 4 cases (36%).

REFERENCES

Aichhorn, A. (1948). *Wayward Youth*. New York: Viking Press.

American Psychiatric Association. (1952). *Diagnostic and Statistical Manual of Mental Disorders*. Washington, D.C.

_____. (1968). *Diagnostic and Statistical Manual*, 2nd Ed. Washington, D.C.

_____. (1977). *Diagnostic and Statistical Manual*, 3rd Ed. Draft Version. New York.

Anthony, E. J. (1958). An aetiological approach to the diagnosis of psychoses in childhood. *Revue de Psychiatrie Infantile* 25:89-96.

_____. (1968). The developmental precursors of adult schizophrenia. *Journal of Psychiatric Research* 6:293-316.

_____. (1969). The reactions of adults to adolescents and their behavior. In G. Caplan and S. Lebovici, Eds., *Adolescence: Psychosocial Perspectives*. New York: Basic Books.

_____. (1970). Two contrasting types of adolescent depression and their treatment. *Journal of the American Psychoanalytic Association* 18:841-859.

_____. (1971). A clinical and experimental study of high-risk children and their schizophrenic parents. In A. Kaplan, Ed., *Genetic Factors in Schizophrenia*. Springfield, Ill.: Thomas.

Arthur, A. Z. (1969). Diagnostic testing and the new alternatives. *Psychological Bulletin* 72:183-192.

Ausubel, D. and Sullivan, E. (1970). *Theory and Problems of Child Development*. New York: Grune & Stratton.

Baldwin, A. L. (1960). The study of child behavior and development. In P. H. Mussen, Ed., *Handbook of Research Methods in Child Development*. New York: Wiley.

Baldwin, A. L., Kalhorn, J. and Breese, F. H. (1949). Patterns of parent behavior. *Psychological Monographs* 63:No. 4.

Bayley, N. (1940). Factors influencing the growth of intelligence in young children. In G. M. Whipple, *Thirty-ninth Yearbook, National Society for the Study of Education*. Bloomington, Ill.: Public School Publishing.

Bender, L. (1947). Childhood schizophrenia. *American Journal of Orthopsychiatry* 17:40-56.

_____. (1953). Childhood schizophrenia *Psychiatric Quarterly* 27:663-668.

_____. (1956). Schizophrenia in childhood—its recognition, description and treatment. *American Journal of Orthopsychiatry* 26:499-506.

_____. (1969). A longitudinal study of schizophrenic children with autism. *Hospital and Community Psychiatry* 20:230-237.

————. (1971). Alpha and omega of childhood schizophrenia. *Journal of Autism and Childhood Schizophrenia* **1**:115-118.

Bender, L. (1973). The lifecourse of children with schizophrenia. *American Journal of Psychiatry* **130**:783-786.

Beres, D. (1958). Vicissitudes of superego function and superego precursors in childhood. *The Psychoanalytic Study of the Child* **13**:324-351. New York: International Universities Press.

————. (1971). Ego autonomy and ego pathology. *The Psychoanalytic Study of the Child* **26**:3-24. New York: International Universities Press.

Birren, J. E. (1944). Psychological examination of children who later became psychotic. *Journal of Abnormal and Social Psychology* **39**:84-96.

Blatt, D. O. and Starr, D. A. (1977). A thriving mini-clinic in a school setting. *Social Casework* **58**:585-595.

Blos, P. (1963). The concept of acting out in relation to the adolescent process. *Journal of the American Academy of Child Psychiatry* **2**:118-136.

————. (1967). The second individuation process of adolescence. *The Psychoanalytic Study of the Child* **22**:162-186. New York: International Universities Press.

————. (1968). Character formation in adolescence. *The Psychoanalytic Study of the Child* **23**:245-263. New York: International Universities Press.

————. (1972). The epigenesis of the adult neurosis. *The Psychoanalytic Study of the Child* **27**:106-135. New York: International Universities Press.

Bomberg, D., Szurek, S. and Etemad, J. (1973). A statistical study of a group of psychotic children. In S. Szurek and I. Berlin, Eds., *Clinical Studies in Childhood Psychoses*. New York: Brunner/Mazel.

Bower, E. M. (1960). *Early Identification of Emotionally Handicapped Children in School*. Springfield, Ill.: Thomas.

Bower, E. M. and Shellhammer, T. D. (1960). School characteristics of male adolescents who later became schizophrenic. *American Journal of Orthopsychiatry* **30**:712-729.

Bowlby, J. (1960). Separation anxiety. *International Journal of Psychoanalysis* **41**:89-113.

Breger, L. (1968). Psychological testing: Treatment and research implications. *Journal of Consulting and Clinical Psychology* **32**:176-181.

Brody, E. (1975). Adolescents as a United States minority group in an era of social change. In A. Esman, Ed., *The Psychology of Adolescence*. New York: International Universities Press.

Bronner, A. (1944). Treatment and what happened afterward. *American Journal of Orthopsychiatry* **14**:28-35.

Brown, J. (1960). Prognosis from presenting symptoms of pre-school children with atypical development. *American Journal of Orthopsychiatry* **30**:382-390.

Brown, J. L. (1969). Adolescent development in children with infantile psychosis. *Seminars in Psychiatry* **1**:79-89.

Cartwright, R. and Vogel, J. (1960). A comparison of changes in psychoneurotic patients during matched periods of therapy and no therapy. *Journal of Consulting Psychology* **24**:121-127.

Cass, L. (1967). Psychotherapy with the obsessive-compulsive child. In M. Hammer and A. Kaplan, eds., *The Practice of Psychotherapy with Children*. Homewood, Ill.: Dorsey.

Clarke, A. M. and Clarke, A. D. B. (1976). *Early Experience: Myth and Evidence*. New York: Free Press.

Cohen, J. (1968). Multiple regression as a general data-analytic system. *Psychological Bulletin* 70:426-443.

Collidge, J. C., Brodie, R. D. and Feeney, B. (1964). A ten-year follow-up study of sixty-six school phobic children. *American Journal of Orthopsychiatry* 34:675-689.

Cooper, S. and Wanerman, L. (1977). *Children in Treatment: A Primer for Beginning Psychotherapists*. New York: Brunner/Mazel.

Cowen, E. L., Pederson, A., Babigian, H. et al. (1973). Long-term follow-up of early detected vulnerable children. *Journal of Consulting and Clinical Psychology* 41:438-446.

Cramer, J. (1959). Common neuroses of childhood. In S. Arieti, Ed., *American Handbook of Psychiatry, 1st Ed.* Vol. I. New York: Basic Books.

Crandall, V. (1972). The Fels study: Some contributions to personality development and achievement in childhood and adulthood. *Seminars in Psychiatry* 4:383-397.

Currie, S., Holtzman, W. and Swartz, J. (1974). Early indicators of personality traits viewed retrospectively. *Journal of School Psychology* 12:51-59.

Davids, A. (1972). *Abnormal Children and Youth: Therapy and Research*. New York: Wiley.

_____, and Salvatore, P. (1976). Residential treatment of disturbed children and adequacy of their subsequent adjustment: A follow-up study. *American Journal of Orthopsychiatry* 46:62-73.

Despert, L. (1955). Differential diagnosis between obsessive-compulsive neurosis and schizophrenia in children. In B. Hoch and J. Zubin, Eds., *Psychopathology of Childhood*. New York: Grune & Stratton.

Edwards, A. S. and Langley, L. D. (1936). Childhood manifestations and adult psychosis. *American Journal of Orthopsychiatry* 6:103-109.

Eiduson, B. T. (1968). Retreat from help. *American Journal of Orthopsychiatry* 38:910-921.

Eisenberg, L. (1957). The course of childhood schizophrenia. *Archives of Neurology and Psychiatry* 78:69-83.

_____. (1972). The classification of childhood psychosis reconsidered. *Journal of Autism and Childhood Schizophrenia* 2:338-342.

_____, and Kanner, L. (1956). Early infantile autism. *American Journal of Orthopsychiatry* 26:556-566.

Ekstein, R. and Wallerstein, J. (1954). Observations on the psychology of borderline and psychotic children. *The Psychoanalytic Study of the Child* 9:344-369. New York: International Universities Press.

Erikson, E. (1950). *Childhood and Society*. New York: Norton.

_____. (1956). The concept of ego identity. *Journal of the American Psychoanalytic Association* 4:56-121.

Erikson, E. (1959) *Identity and the Life Cycle*. New York: International Universities Press.

Escalona, S. and Herder, G. M. (1959). *Prediction and Outcome*. New York: Basic Books.

Esman, A. (1975). *The Psychology of Adolescence*. New York: International Universities Press.

Etemad, J. G. and Szurek, S. A. (1973). A modified follow-up study of a group of psychotic children. In S. Szurek and I. Berlin, Eds., *Clinical Studies in Childhood Psychosis*. New York: Brunner/Mazel.

Fenichel, O. (1945). *The Psychoanalytic Theory of Neurosis*. New York: Norton.

Field, H. (1969). Prediction of character disorder and psychotic outcome from childhood behavior. Unpublished Thesis, New York, Teacher's College, Columbia University.

Fischer, J. (1976). *The Effectiveness of Social Casework*. Springfield, Ill.: Thomas.

Fraiberg, S. (1969). Libidinal object constancy and mental representation. *The Psychoanalytic Study of the Child* 24:9-47. New York: International Universities Press.

Frank, L. K. (1963). Human development: An emerging scientific discipline. In A. Solnit and S. Provence, Eds., *Modern Perspectives in Child Development*. New York: International Universities Press.

Frazee, H. E. (1953). Children who later became schizophrenic. *Smith College Studies in Social Work* 23:125-149.

Freud, A. (1942). *The Ego and the Mechanisms of Defense*. London: Hogarth.

———. (1952). Mutual influence in the development of ego and id. *The Psychoanalytic Study of the Child* 7:42-50. New York: International Universities Press.

———. (1958a). Adolescence. *The Psychoanalytic Study of the Child* 13:255-278. New York: International Universities Press.

———. (1958b). Child observation and prediction of development: A memorial lecture in honor of Ernest Kris. *The Psychoanalytic Study of the Child* 13:92-124. New York: International Universities Press.

———. (1962). Assessment of childhood disturbances. *The Psychoanalytic Study of the Child* 17:149-158. New York: International Universities Press.

———. (1963). The concept of developmental lines. *The Psychoanalytic Study of the Child* 18:245-265. New York: International Universities Press.

———. (1965). *Normality and Pathology in Childhood*. New York: International Universities Press.

———. (1969). Research at the Hampstead Child-Therapy Clinic and Other Papers. In *Writings of Anna Freud*, V. New York: International Universities Press.

———. (1972). The infantile neurosis: Genetic and dynamic considerations. *The Psychoanalytic Study of the Child* 26:78-89. New York: International Universities Press.

———. (1977). Assessment of childhood disturbances. In R. Essler, A. Freud, M. Kris, and A. Solnit, Eds., *Psychoanalytic Assessment: The Diagnostic Profile*. New Haven: Yale University Press.

Freud, S. (1955a). Analysis of a phobia in a five-year old boy (1909). In *Standard Edition of the Complete Psychological Works of Sigmund Freud*, X. London: Hogarth.

_____. (1955b). The psychogenesis of a case of homosexuality in a woman (1920). In *Standard Edition of the Complete Psychological Works of Sigmund Freud*, XVIII. London: Hogarth.

_____. (1958). The disposition to obsessional neurosis (1913). In *Standard Edition of the Complete Psychological Works of Sigmund Freud*, XII. London: Hogarth.

_____. (1961a). The future of an illusion (1927). In *Standard Edition of the Complete Psychological Works of Sigmund Freud*, XXI. London: Hogarth.

_____. (1961b). The ego and the id (1923). In *Standard Edition of the Complete Psychological Works of Sigmund Freud*, XIX. London: Hogarth.

_____. (1961c). Civilization and its discontents (1930). In *Standard Edition of the Complete Psychological Works of Sigmund Freud*, XXI. London: Hogarth.

Gardner, G. (1967). The relationship between childhood neurotic symptomatology and later schizophrenia in males and females. *Journal of Nervous and Mental Disease* 144:97-100.

Garmezy, N. (1971). Vulnerability research and the issue of primary prevention. *American Journal of Orthopsychiatry* 41:101-116.

Geleerd, E. R. (1958). Borderline states in childhood and adolescence. *The Psychoanalytic Study of the Child* 13:279-295. New York: International Universities Press.

Gersten, J. C., Langner, T. S. and Eisenberg, J. D. (1976). Stability and change in types of behavioral disturbance in children and adolescents. *Journal of Abnormal Child Psychology* 4:111-127.

Gildea, M. C.-L., Glidewell, J. C. and Kantor, M. B. (1967). The St. Louis School mental health project: History and evaluation. In E. Cowen, E. Gardner and M. Zax, Eds., *Emergent Approach to Mental Health Problems*. New York: Appleton-Century-Crofts.

Glasscote, R. M., Fishman, M., and Sonis, M. (1972). *Children and Mental Health Centers*. Washington, D.C.: Joint Information Service.

_____. Sanders, D., Forstenzer, K. M., and Foley, A. R. (1964). *The Community Mental Health Center*. Baltimore: Garamond Pridemark.

Glidewell, J. C., Gildea, M. C.-L., Domke, H. R. and Kantor, M. B. (1959). Behavior symptoms in children and adjustment in public school. *Human Organization* 18(3):123-130.

_____, Mensh, I. and Gildea, M. C.-L. (1957) Behavior symptoms in children and degree of sickness. *American Journal of Psychiatry* 114(1):47-53.

Glueck, S., and Glueck, E. (1940). *Juvenile Delinquents Grown Up*. New York: The Commonwealth Fund.

_____. (1959). *Predicting Delinquency and Crime*. Cambridge: Harvard University Press.

Goldfarb, W. (1970). A follow-up investigation of schizophrenic children treated in residence. *Psychosocial Process, Journal of Jewish Board of Guardians* 1:1.

_____. (1972). An investigation of childhood schizophrenia: A retrospective review.

In S. Harrison and J. McDermott, Eds., *Childhood Psychopathology*. New York: International Universities Press.

Goldstein, J. and Rodnick, E. H. (1975). The family contribution to the etiology of schizophrenia: Current status. *Schizophrenia Bulletin* **14**:48-63.

Graham, P., Rutter, M. and George, S. (1973). Temperamental characteristics as predictors of behavior disorders in children. *American Journal of Orthopsychiatry* **43**:328-339.

Group for the Advancement of Psychiatry. (1966). *Psychopathological Disorders in Childhood: Theoretical Considerations and a Proposed Classification.* GAP Report No. 62.

Haan, N. (1972). Personality development from adolescence to adulthood in the Oakland growth and guidance studies. *Seminars in Psychiatry* **4**:399-414.

Harrison, S. I. and McDermott, J. F. (1972). *Childhood Psychopathology.* New York: International Universities Press.

Hartmann, H. (1950). Comments on the psychoanalytic theory of the ego. *The Psychoanalytic Study of the Child* **5**:74-96. New York: International Universities Press.

————. (1952). Mutual influences in the development of ego and id. *The Psychoanalytic Study of the Child*, **7**:9-30. New York: International Universities Press.

————. (1953). Contributions to the metapsychology of schizophrenia. *The Psychoanalytic Study of the Child* **8**:177-197. New York: International Universities Press.

————, Kris, E., and Lowenstein, R. M. (1946). Comments on the formation of psychic structure. *The Psychoanalytic Study of the Child*, **2**:11-37. New York: International Universities Press.

Havelkova, M. (1968). Follow-up study of 71 children diagnosed as psychotic in preschool age. *American Journal of Orthopsychiatry* **38**:846-857.

Havighurst, R. M., Bowman, P. H., Liddle, G. P. et al. (1962). *Growing Up in River City.* New York: Wiley.

Healy, W. and Bronner, A. F. (1936). *New Light on Delinquency and its Treatment.* New Haven: Yale University Press.

Heinicke, C. M. (1969). Frequency of psychotherapeutic session as a factor affecting outcome. Analysis of clinical ratings and test results. *Journal of Abnormal Psychology* **74**:553-560.

————. (1976). Aiding at risk children through psychoanalytic social work with parents. *American Journal of Orthopsychiatry* **46**:89-103.

————, and Goldman, A. (1960). Research on psychotherapy with children: A review and suggestions for further study. *American Journal of Orthopsychiatry* **30**:483-494.

————, and Strassman, L. H. (1975). Toward more effective research on child psychotherapy. *Journal of the American Academy of Child Psychiatry* **14**:561-588.

Hersch, C. (1968). The discontent explosion in mental health. *American Psychologist* **23**:497-506.

Hunt, J. V. and Eichorn, D. H. (1972). Maternal and child behaviors: A review of data from the Berkeley Growth Study. *Seminars in Psychiatry* **4**:367-381.

Jacobson, E. (1954). The self and the object world. *The Psychoanalytic Study of the Child* **9**:75-127. New York: International Universities Press.

_____. (1957). Denial and repression. *Journal of the American Psychoanalytic Association* **5**:61-92.

Janes, C. L. and Hesselbrock, V. M. (1978). Problem children's adjustment predicted from teachers' ratings. *American Journal of Orthopsychiatry* **48**:300-309.

Jenkins, R. L. (1960). The psychopathic or antisocial personality. *Journal of Nervous and Mental Disease* **131**:318-334.

Joint Commission on Mental Health of Children (1969). *Report.* Washington, D.C.

_____. 1961. *Action for Mental Health.* New York: Basic Books.

Jones, M. C., Bayley, N., Macfarlane, J. W. and Honzek, M. P. (1971). *The Course of Human Development.* Waltham, Mass.: Xerox College Publishing.

Josselyn, I. M. (1952). *The Adolescent and His World.* New York: Family Service Association of America.

Kagan, J. (1964). American longitudinal research on psychological development. Child Development **35**:1-32.

_____. (1976). Resilience and continuity in psychological development. In A. M. Clarke and A. D. B. Clarke, Eds., *Early Experience: Myth and Evidence.* New York: Free Press.

_____, and Moss, H. A. (1962). *Birth to Maturity.* New York: Wiley.

Kanfer, F. N. and Saslow, G. (1965). Behavioral analysis. *Archives of General Psychiatry* **12**:529-539.

_____. (1969). Behavioral diagnosis. In C. Franks, Ed., *Assessment and Status of the Behavioral Therapies and Associated Developments.* New York: McGraw-Hill.

Kanner, L. (1943). Autistic disturbances of affective contact. *Nervous Child* **2**:217-250.

_____. (1949). Problems of nosology and psychodynamics of early autism. *American Journal of Orthopsychiatry* **19**:416-426.

_____. (1952). The conception of whole and parts in early infantile autism. *American Journal of Psychiatry* **108**:23-26.

_____. (1960). Do behavioral symptoms always indicate psychopathology? *Journal of Child Psychology and Psychiatry* **1**:17-25.

_____, and Eisenberg, L. (1955). Notes on the follow-up studies of autistic children. In B. Hoch and J. Zubin, Eds., *Psychopathology of Childhood.* New York: Grune & Stratton.

Kessler, J. W. (1977). Appendix C. In H. Strupp, S. Hadley and B. Gomes-Schwartz, Eds., *Psychotherapy for Better or Worse.* New York: Jason Aronson.

Klein, M. (1939). *The Psycho-Analysis of Children.* London: Hogarth.

Knight, R. P. (1953). Borderline states. In R. M. Lowenstein, Ed., *Drives, Affects, Behavior.* New York: International Universities Press.

Koch, E. (1973). Observations on follow-up contact with former child analytic patients. *Journal of the American Academy of Child Psychiatry* **12**:223-246.

Kohlberg, L., LaCrosse, J. and Ricks, D. (1972). The predictability of adult mental health from childhood behavior. In B. Wolman, Ed., *Manual of Child Psychopathology*. New York: McGraw-Hill.

Kolvin, I., Ounsted, C., Humphrey, M. and McNay, D. (1971). The phenomenology of childhood psychosis. *British Journal of Psychiatry* **118**:385-395.

Kolvin, I. et al. (1971). Studies in the childhood psychoses. *British Journal of Psychiatry* **118**:381-419.

Kris, E. (1950). Notes on the development and on some current problems of psychoanalytic child psychology. *The Psychoanalytic Study of the Child* **5**:24-46. New York: International Universities Press.

Kupfer, D. J., Detre, T. P. and Koral, J. (1975). Relationship of certain childhood "traits" to adult psychiatric disorders. *American Journal of Orthopsychiatry* **45**:74-81.

Langner, H. P. (1971). The making of a murderer. *American Journal of Psychiatry* **127**:950-953.

Lapouse, R. and Monk, M. A. (1958). An epidemiologic study of behavior characteristics in children. *American Journal of Public Health* **48**:1134.

Lehrman, L. S., Sirluck, H., Black, B. J. and Glick, S. (1949). Success and failure of treatment of children in the Child Guidance Clinics of the Jewish Board of Guardians. *New York City Jewish Board of Guardians, Research Monograph*, No. 1.

Lessing, E. E. and Schilling, F. H. (1966). Relationship between treatment selection variables and treatment outcome in a child guidance clinic. *Journal of the American Academy of Child Psychiatry* **5**:313-347.

Leventhal, T. and Weinberger, G. (1975). Evaluation of a large-scale brief therapy program for children. *American Journal of Orthopsychiatry* **45**:119-132.

Levitt, E. E. (1957). The results of psychotherapy with children: An evaluation. *Journal of Consulting Psychology* **21**:189-195.

————. (1963). Psychotherapy with children. *Behaviour Research and Therapy Quarterly* **1**:45-51.

————. (1971). Research on psychotherapy with children. In A. Berger and S. Garfield, Eds., *Handbook of Psychotherapy and Behavior Change*. New York: Wiley.

Levy, E. Z. (1969). Long-term follow-up of former inpatients at the Children's Hospital of the Menninger Clinic. *American Journal of Psychiatry* **125**:633-639.

Lewis, S. B., Barnhart, F. D., Gosset, J. T., and Phillips, V. A. (1975). Follow-up of adolescents treated in a psychiatric hospital. *American Journal of Orthopsychiatry* **45**:813-824.

Lewis, W. W. (1965). Continuity and intervention in emotional disturbance: A review. *Exceptional Children* **31**:465-475.

Livson, N. and Peskin, H. (1967). Prediction of adult psychological health in a longitudinal study. *Journal of Abnormal and Social Psychology* **72**:509-515.

Lo, W. H. (1973). A note on a follow-up study of childhood neurosis and behavior disorder. *Journal of Child Psychology and Psychiatry* **14**:147-150.

Lotter, V. (1974). Social adjustment and placement of autistic children in Middlesex: A follow-up study. *Journal of Autism and Childhood Schizophrenia* **4**:11-32.

Love, L. and Kaswan, J. (1974). *Troubled Children: Their Families, Schools and Treatment.* New York: Wiley.

Macfarlane, J., Allen, L. and Honzik, M. (1954). *A Developmental Study of the Behavior Problems of Normal Children.* Berkeley: University of California Press.

Maenchen, A. (1953). Notes on early ego disturbances. *The Psychoanalytic Study of the Child* **8**:177-197. New York: International Universities Press.

Mahler, M. S. (1952). On child psychosis and schizophrenia: Autistic and symbiotic infantile psychoses. *The Psychoanalytic Study of the Child* **7**:286-305. New York: International Universities Press.

_____. (1963). Thoughts about development and individuation. *The Psychoanalytic Study of the Child* **18**:307-324. New York: International Universities Press.

_____, and Furer, M. (1972). Child psychosis: A theoretical statement and its implications. *Journal of Autism and Childhood Schizophrenia* **2**:213-218.

Marceil, J. C. (1977). Implicit dimensions of idiography and nomothesis: A reformulation. *American Psychologist* **32**:1046-1055.

Masterson, J. E. (1967a). *The Psychiatric Dilemma of Adolescence.* Boston: Little, Brown.

_____. (1967b). The symptomatic adolescent five years later: He didn't grow out of it. *American Journal of Psychiatry* **123**:1338-1345.

_____. (1968). The psychiatric significance of adolescent turmoil. *American Journal of Psychiatry* **124**: 1549-1554.

McGarrity, M. (1975). Building early relationships in school social work. *Social Casework* **56**:323-327.

McLaughlin, B. E. (1965). *Long-Term Results of Psychiatric Out-Patient Treatment.* Springfield, Ill.: Thomas.

Mead, M. (1930). Adolescence in primitive and modern society. In V. Calverton and S. Schmalhausen, Eds., *The New Generation.* New York: Maccaulay.

Mednick, S. A. and McNeil, T. F. (1968) Current methodology in research on the etiology of schizophrenia: Serious difficulties which suggest the use of the high-risk group method. *Psychological Bulletin* **70**:681-693.

_____, and Schulsinger, F. (1970) Factors related to breakdown in children at high risk for schizophrenia. In M. Roff and D. Ricks, Eds., *Life History Research in Psychopathology* **1**:51-93. Minneapolis: University of Minnesota Press.

Meehl, P. E. (1954). *Clinical vs. Statistical Prediction.* Minneapolis: University of Minnesota Press.

Mellsop, G. (1972). Psychiatric patients seen as children and adults: Childhood predictors of adult illness. *Journal of Child Psychology and Psychiatry* **13**:91-101.

Meltzoff, J. and Kornreich, M. (1970). *Research in Psychotherapy.* New York: Atherton Press.

Menolascino, F. and Eaton, L. (1968). Psychoses of childhood. A five-year follow-up of experiences in a mental retardation clinic." In S. Chess and A. Thomas, Eds., *Annual Progress in Child Psychiatry and Child Development.* New York: Brunner/Mazel.

Meyer, J. and Zegans, L. (1975). Adolescents perceive their psychotherapy. *Psychiatry* **38**:11-22.

Michael, C. M., Morris, D. and Soroker, E. (1957). Follow-up studies of shy withdrawn children, II. Relative incidence of schizophrenia. *American Journal of Orthopsychiatry* **27**:331-337.

Mitchell, J. C. (1949). A study of teachers' and of mental hygienists' rating of certain behavior problems in children. *Journal of Educational Research* **39**:292-307.

Morris, D., Soroker, E., and Burruss, G. (1954). Follow-up studies of shy, withdrawn children, I. Evaluation of later adjustment. *American Journal of Orthopsychiatry* **24**:743-754.

Morris, H. H. Jr., Escoll, P. J. and Wexler, R. (1956). Aggressive behavior disorders of childhood: A follow-up study. *American Journal of Psychiatry* **112**:991-997.

Murphy, L. B. and Moriarty, A. E. (1976). *Vulnerability, Coping and Growth.* New Haven: Yale University Press.

National Institute of Mental Health, (1973a). U.S. Department of Health, Education and Welfare, Series B, No. 5 Utilization of mental health facilities. *Analytical and Special Study Reports.*

————. (1973b). Utilization of psychiatric facilities by persons under 18 years of age. *Mental Health Statistical Note*, No. 90.

————. (1976). *Mental Health Statistical Note*, No. 127: Provisional data on patient case episodes in mental health facilities.

Offer, D. (1969). Adolescent turmoil. In A. Esman, Ed., *The Psychological World of the Teen-ager: A Study of Normal Adolescent Boys.* New York: Basic Books.

Offord, D. R. and Cross, L. A. (1969). Behavioral antecedents of adult schizophrenia. A review. *Archives of General Psychiatry* **21**:207-283.

O'Neal, P. and Robins, L. N. (1958). Childhood patterns predictive of adult schizophrenia: A 30-year follow-up study. *American Journal of Psychiatry* **115**:385-391.

Pearson, G. (1949). *Emotional Disorders of Children.* New York: Norton.

Peskin, H. (1972). Multiple prediction of adult psychological health from preadolescent and adolescent behavior. *Journal of Consulting and Clinical Psychology* **38**:155.

————, and Livson, N. (1972). Pre- and postpubertal personality and adult psychologic functioning. *Seminars in Psychiatry* **4**:343-353.

Piggott, L. R. and Gottlieb, J. S. (1974). Childhood schizophrenia—What is it? In S. Chess and A. Thomas, Eds., *Annual Progress in Child Psychiatry and Child Development.* New York: Brunner/Mazel.

Pollack, M., Levenstein, S., and Klein, D. (1968). A three-year post-hospital follow-up of adolescent and adult schizophrenics. *American Journal of Orthopsychiatry* **38**:94-109.

————, Woerner, M. G., Goodman, W. and Greenberg, I. W. (1966). Childhood development patterns of hospitalized adult schizophrenic and nonschizophrenic patients and their siblings. *American Journal of Orthopsychiatry* **36**:510-517.

Rachman, S. (1971). *The Effects of Psychotherapy.* New York: Pergamon Press.

Redl, F. and Wineman, D. (1951). *Children Who Hate.* New York: Free Press.

Ricks, D. F. (1974). Supershrink: Methods of a therapist judged successful on the basis of adult outcomes of adolescent patients. In D. Ricks, A. Thomas and M. Roff, Eds., *Life History Research in Psychotherapy,* Vol. III. Minneapolis: University of Minnesota Press.

Riddle, K. D. and Rapoport, J. L. (1976). A 2-year follow-up of 72 hyperactive boys. *Journal of Nervous and Mental Disease* 162:126-133.

Ridenour, N. (1961). *Mental Health in the United States: A Fifty Year History.* Cambridge, Mass.: Harvard University Press.

Robins, L. N. (1966). *Deviant Children Grown Up.* Baltimore: Williams & Wilkins.

_____. (1972). Follow-up studies of behavior disorders in children. In H. C. Quay and J. S. Werry, Eds., *Psychopathological Disorders of Childhood.* New York: Wiley.

_____, and O'Neal, P. (1958). Mortality, mobility and crime: Problem children thirty years later. *American Sociological Review* 23:162-171.

Rodriguez, A., Rodriguez, M., and Eisenberg, L. (1960). The outcome of school phobia: A follow-up based on 41 cases. *American Journal of psychiatry* 116: 540-544.

Roff, J. D., Knight, R. and Wertheim, E. (1976). Disturbed preschizophrenics, childhood symptoms in relation to adult outcome. *Journal of Nervous and Mental Disease* 162:274-281.

Roff, M. (1974). Childhood antecedents of adult neurosis, severe bad conduct and psychological health. *Life History Research in Psychopathology* 3:131-162.

Rogers, C. R. (1942). Mental health findings in three elementary schools. *Educational Research Bulletin* 21:69-79.

Rosenfeld, S. K. and Sprince, M. P. (1963). An attempt to formulate the meaning of the concept 'borderline.' *The Psychoanalytic Study of the Child* 18:603-635. New York: International Universities Press.

Rosenthal, A. and Levine, S. (1970). Brief psychotherapy with children: A preliminary report. *American Journal of Psychiatry* 127:646-651.

Rosenzweig, S. (1958). The place of the individual and of idiodynamics in psychology: A dialogue. *Journal of Individual Psychology* 14:3-21.

Ross, A. O. and Lacey, H. M. (1961). Characteristics of terminators and remainers in child guidance treatment. *Journal of Consulting Psychology* 25:420-424.

Rutter, M. (1972). Childhood schizophrenia reconsidered. *Journal of Autism and Childhood Schizophrenia* 2:315-337.

_____. (1975). *Helping Troubled Children.* New York: Plenum Press.

_____. (1976). Parent-child separation: Psychological effects on the children. In A. M. Clarke and A. D. B. Clarke, Eds., *Early Experience: Myth and Evidence.* New York: Free Press.

_____, Greenfeld, D. and Lockyer, L. (1968). A five to fifteen year follow-up study of infantile psychoses. In S. Chess and A. Thomas, Eds., *Annual Progress in Child Psychiatry and Child Development.* New York: Brunner/Mazel.

Sahakian, W. S., Ed. (1965). *Psychology of Pesonality: Readings in Theory*. Chicago: Rand McNally.

Sargent, H., Horwitz, L., Wallerstein, R. and Appelbaum, A. (1968). *Prediction in Psychotherapy Research: A Method for the Transformation of Clinical Judgments into Testable Hypothesis*. New York: International Universities Press.

Schacht, T., and Nathan, P. (1977). But is it good for the psychologists? Appraisal and status of DSM-III. *American Psychologist* 32:1017-1025.

Schofield, W. and Balian, L. (1959). A comparative study of the personal histories of schizophrenic and nonpsychiatric patients. *Journal of Abnormal and Social Psychology* 59:216-225.

Settlage, C. F. (1964). Psychologic disorders. In W. E. Nelson, Ed., *Textbook of Pediatrics,* 8th Ed. Philadelphia: Saunders.

Shaffer, D. (1974). Psychiatric aspects of brain injury in childhood: A review. In S. Chess and A. Thomas, Eds., *Annual Progress in Child Psychiatry and Child Development*. New York: Brunner/Mazel.

Shepherd, M., Oppenheim, A. N. and Mitchell, S. (1966). Childhood behavior disorders and the child-guidance clinic: An epidemiological study. *Journal of Child Psychology and Psychiatry* 7:39-52.

Shore, M. and Massimo, J. (1973). After ten years: A follow-up study of comprehensive vocationally oriented psychotherapy. *American Journal of Orthopsychiatry* 43:128-134.

Silverman, J. S. and Ross, N. (1972). Mental disorders in childhood and adolescence. In B. Wolman, Ed., *Handbook of Child Psychoanalysis*. New York: Van Nostrand Reinhold.

Sindberg, R. M. (1970) A fifteen year follow-up study of community guidance clinic clients. *Community Mental Health* 6:319-324.

Skeels, H. M. and Skodak M. (1965). Techniques for a high-yield follow-up study in the field. *Public Health Reports* 80:249-257.

Speer, D. C. (1971). Behavior problem checklist (Peterson-Quay): Baseline data from parents of child guidance and non-clinic children. *Journal of Consulting and Clinical Psychology* 36:221-228.

Srole, L., Langner, T. S. and Michael, S. T. (1962). *Mental Health in the Metropolis: The Midtown Manhattan Study*, Vol. 1. New York: McGraw-Hill.

Stabenau, J. and Pollen, W. (1970). Comparative life history differences of families of schizophrenics, delinquents and "normals." In M. Roff and D. Ricks, Eds., *Life History Research in Psychopathology* I. Minneapolis: University of Minnesota Press.

Stenneth, R. G. (1966). Emotional handicap in the elementary school years: Phase or disease? *American Journal of Orthopsychiatry* 36:444-449.

Strupp, H. and Hadley, S. (1977). A tripartite model of mental health and therapeutic outcomes: With special reference to negative effects in psychotherapy. *American Psychologist* 32:187-196.

Stuart, R. B. (1970). *Trick or Treatment: How and When Psychotherapy Fails*. Champaign, Ill.: Research Press.

Thomas, A. and Chess, S. (1976). Evolution of behavior disorders into adolescence. *American Journal of Psychiatry* **133**:539-542.

_____. (1977). *Temperament and Development.* New York: Brunner/Mazel.

_____, and Birch, H. (1968). *Temperament and Behavior Disorders in Children.* New York: New York University Press.

Ullman, C. (1952a). Identification of maladjusted school children. *Public Health Monograph*, No. 7.

_____. (1952b). Mental health screening of school children. *Public Health Reports, U.S. Department of Health, Education and Welfare* **67**:1219-1223.

_____. (1957). Teachers, peers and tests as predictors of adjustment. *Journal of Educational Psychology* **48**:257-267.

Waldron, S. (1976). The significance of childhood neurosis for adult mental health. *American Journal of Psychiatry* **133**:532-538.

Watt, N. F. (1972). Longitudinal changes in the social behavior of children hospitalized for schizophrenia as adults. *Journal of Nervous and Mental Disease* **155**:42-54.

_____, Stolorow, R. D., Lubensky, A. and McClelland, D. (1970). School adjustment and behavior of children hospitalized for schizophrenia as adults. *American Journal of Orthopsychiatry* **40**:637-657.

Weil, A. (1953). Certain severe disturbances of ego development in childhood. *The Psychoanalytic Study of the Child* **8**:271-287. New York: International Universities Press.

Weiss, M. and Burke, A. (1970). A five- to ten-year follow up of hospitalized school phobic children and adolescents. *American Journal of Orthopsychiatry* **40**:672-676.

Whittaker, J. K. (1976). Causes of childhood disorder. New findings. *Social Work* **21**:91-96.

Wickman, E. K. (1928). *Children's Behavior and Teacher's Attitudes.* New York: Commonwealth Fund.

Wimberger, H. C. and Millar, G. (1968). The psychotherapeutic effects of initial clinic contact on child psychiatry patients. In S. Lesse, Ed., *An Evaluation of the Results of the Psychotherapies.* Springfield, Ill.: Thomas.

Witmer, H. and Keller, J. (1942). Outgrowing childhood problems: A study of the value of child guidance treatment. *Smith College Studies in Social Work* **13**:74-90.

Wolman, B. (1970). Childhood schizophrenia or vectoriasis praecocissima. *American Journal of Psychotherapy* **24**:264-277.

_____. (1972). *Handbook of Child Psychoanalysis: Research Theory and Practice.* New York: Van Nostrand Reinhold.

Zold, A. and Speer, D. (1971). Follow-up study of child guidance clinic patients by means of the behavior problems checklist. *Journal of Clinical Psychology* **27**:519-524.

Author Index

Subject Index